SHORT LOAN

5000591072

University of Hertfordshire

ROYAL MILITARY COLLEGE

Please return on or before the last date stamped below.

1 6 MAY 1996
1 1 NOV 1999

Repro C195

 WITH

D1428917

ATYPICAL ORTHOPEDIC RADIOGRAPHIC PROCEDURES

ATYPICAL ORTHOPEDIC RADIOGRAPHIC PROCEDURES

GARY L. WATKINS, M.Ed., R.T.(R)

Associate Professor
Department of Radiographic Science
Idaho State University
Pocatello, Idaho

THOMAS F. MOORE, M.Ed., R.T.(R)

Assistant Professor
Department of Radiographic Science
Idaho State University
Pocatello, Idaho

With **155** *illustrations*

ROYAL MILITARY COLLEGE OF SCIENCE
LIBRARY

Control No.....................

Class No......617.3.141.WAT

Date Received -.5 OCT 1995

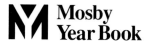

Mosby
Year Book

St. Louis   Baltimore   Boston   Chicago   London   Philadelphia   Sydney   Toronto

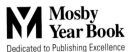

Mosby
Year Book
Dedicated to Publishing Excellence

Publisher: David T. Culverwell
Editorial Project Supervisor: Cecilia F. Reilly
Project Manager: Annette Hall
Designer: Gail Morey Hudson

Copyright © 1993 by Mosby–Year Book, Inc.
A Mosby imprint of Mosby–Year Book, Inc.

All rights reserved. No part of this publication may be reproduced, stored in a retrieval system, or transmitted, in any form or by any means, electronic, mechanical, photocopying, recording, or otherwise, without prior written permission from the publisher.

Permission to photocopy or reproduce solely for internal or personal use is permitted for libraries or other users registered with the Copyright Clearance Center, provided that the base fee of $4.00 per chapter plus $.10 per page is paid directly to the Copyright Clearance Center, 27 Congress Street, Salem, MA 01970. This consent does not extend to other kinds of copying, such as copying for general distribution, for advertising or promotional purposes, for creating new collected works, or for resale.

Printed in the United States of America

Mosby–Year Book, Inc.
11830 Westline Industrial Drive
St. Louis, Missouri 63146

Library of Congress Cataloging in Publication Data
Watkins, Gary L.
    Atypical orthopedic radiographic procedures / Gary L. Watkins, Thomas F. Moore.
        p.   cm.
    Includes bibliographical references and index.
    ISBN 0-8016-6270-2
    1. Radiography in orthopedics.   I. Moore, Thomas F.   II. Title.
    [DNLM: 1. Bone and Bones—radiography.   2. Joints—pathology.
    3. Orthopedics—methods.   WE 141 W335a]
RD743.5.R33W38   1993
617.3—dc20
DNLM/DLC
for Library of Congress   92-49255
                                                                  CIP

92 93 94 95 96 CL/VH 9 8 7 6 5 4 3 2 1

To my dear wife
PAULA
G.L.W.

To my
FAMILY
T.F.M.

Preface

This book arises from some of our experiences in the hospital setting. We remember that, all too frequently, either a radiologist or an orthopedic surgeon asked us to perform some atypical orthopedic radiographic procedure which we were certain we had never heard of, much less performed. The physician had a very specific radiographic result in mind and expected us to produce it. We somehow fumbled through these procedures, ultimately producing the desired final result; but we never truly understood what we were doing or why. *Atypical Orthopedic Radiographic Procedures* is aimed at relieving radiographers and physicians of some of this misery.

To arrive at the procedures presented here we requested that radiographers and orthopedic surgeons across the country send us information concerning any atypical orthopedic radiographic procedures which they commonly use. Much to our pleasure and the benefit of the book some radiologists responded to our request also. In addition, we surveyed the radiography and orthopedic surgery literature, both journals and texts, to arrive at the book's final contents. We feel that what is offered here is both unique and valuable, especially for the practitioner who is interested in radiographically imaging a specific body part in order to rule out or better assess a specific pathologic condition.

Although the medical literature was a valuable source for finding these procedures, we found that we had to change some of the terminology used to describe these procedures. Radiography terminology is highly specialized and isn't necessarily always used in descriptions of radiographic projections or positions. We have attempted to present only the most correct terminology in use in radiography which accurately describes how each procedure is accomplished and the anatomy that each procedure is intended to demonstrate.

The primary use for this book is as a reference text for both radiographers and physicians. The radiographer who is faced with a particular orthopedic imaging problem will look to this book for the solution to that problem. Orthopedic surgeons, emergency room physicians, and family practitioners who need to radiographically demonstrate some specific anatomic part to rule out a specific orthopedic condition will also look to this book for the solution. A secondary need as a classroom textbook for the student radiographer is also fulfilled by making the student aware of the realm of imaging possibilities in orthopedic procedures. This book will be of value in one or more radiographic procedures, positioning, or methods courses in radiography programs. It is primarily descriptive and therefore lends itself well to these kinds of courses and laboratory courses. We believe that the student radiographer, the radiographer, and the physician alike will find this an easy-to-use book that will be consulted frequently.

In the first chapter we have explained the special care that the orthopedic patient requires in terms of the possible orthopedic injuries. We also explain some basic considerations for determining the exposure factors and imaging parameters to be used in orthopedic radiography. Orthopedic assessment and treatment are becoming more highly specialized in all facets of medicine, including radiography. These special considerations of the orthopedic patient and orthopedic imaging are becoming increasingly important.

In the remaining chapters we present the procedures in a logical order beginning with the upper limb; progressing through to the shoulder girdle, bony thorax, and lower limb; and concluding with the hip, pelvis, and spine. In addition to accurately describing how each procedure is performed we have indicated the specific orthopedic condition that each procedure is intended to demonstrate. Other uses for each procedure, however, may also exist. For example, we present the "PA 10 Degree Axial" wrist as being valuable to demonstrate scapholunate subluxation. Since we started writing this book, we have found others who have successfully used this same position to demonstrate fractures of the capitate. Radiographs of the intended outcome are presented as are photographs of the patient position to further guide the user to the desired radiographic result. The book is designed to be used expediently and efficiently, thereby increasing its utility. References are provided for most procedures for those who desire more indepth information.

Finally, we have used the word "atypical" in the title of the book, but we believe the use of these procedures is not. We found many of these procedures repeated in many sources and have, whenever possible, referenced the most primary source. We hope that you as the user of this book will agree that the use of the procedures presented here is valuable in your professional practice.

GLW
TFM

Acknowledgments

We would especially like to thank Chuck Francis, Dave Myers, Chari Breiner, and Doug Wehrli. We also gratefully extend our appreciation and gratitude to the following people: M.S. Anderson, Molly Arnzen, Janna Atkins, Ellen Avery, Nicholas Barnes, Dr. Sarah Bowman, Linda Brittain, Dr. Karen Brown, Brent Bywater, Lisa Cameron, Tracy Christensen, James Creelman, Dr. Susan Daleiden, Carrie Davis, Danny Davis, Teri Dickerson, Vicki Dishon, Dr. Allen Eng, Bruce Foster, Gloria Hahn, Monica Hamberlin, Ivana Hanners, Robbie Hansen, Steve Hansen, D. Richelle Harmon, Marlene Hilton, Grace Jacobsen, Greg Kearns, Cheryl Kudla, Cari Larson, Candi Leavitt, Kristi Lords, Dr. J. T. Malouf, Lita McArthur, Linda Meachum, Cristy Mecham, Deb Miller, Dr. William Mott, Brian Myer, Pat Potter, John Reynolds, Kim Robertson, Teresa Ruckman, Sherry Schaefer, Steve Self, Mehran Seyed-Hosseini, Sandra Shaker, Jan Sisler, Marsha Sortor, Cheryl Taylor, Dr. Alex Urfer, David Wetzel, and Lori Wright.

Contents

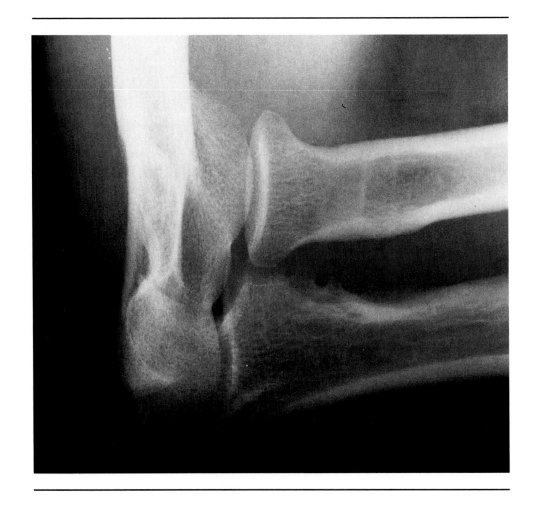

Introduction to Orthopedic Radiography

SPECIAL CARE OF ORTHOPEDIC PATIENTS

Patients with orthopedic injuries or conditions require special care on the part of the radiographer and physician. The extent of the patient's injury can worsen as a result of careless or inappropriate consideration of the patient's condition. Specifically, possible joint injuries, possible fractures, severe trauma, and inflammatory joint diseases require special treatment. Ignorance of this fact may cause practitioners to further injure the patient or exacerbate the condition and compromise the quality of care provided for that patient. It is of the utmost importance that the radiographer and physician take into consideration the type and extent of patient injury or condition before performing any radiographic procedure on that patient.

Patients with Possible Joint Injuries or Conditions

Joint injuries may include dislocations or other less obvious conditions such as ligament injury or inflammatory joint disease. Until the full extent of the patient's injury or condition has been determined, for the purpose of prudent patient care, the radiographer should treat the patient as if a joint injury or condition exists. Patients should always be questioned about the pain they are feeling before any radiographic procedure is begun. Radiographic procedures that necessitate the movement of an injured or inflamed joint may exacerbate the injury or condition of that joint; this movement should always be done with caution. Radiographic procedures must be selected with the possibility of joint injury or inflammation in mind. If the patient seems unable to move the joint in question or exhibits pain while doing so, the radiographer should consult the physician concerning the radiographs to be produced. No patient should be forced into a radiographic position if it is obviously painful to move into that position. The physician, in consultation with the radiogra-

1

pher, should be the only person to decide if the radiographic procedure should be completed based on the condition of the patient.

Some radiographic procedures used to assess joint injury require that the joint be stressed. Joint injuries may be accompanied by fracture, and stressing a joint may exacerbate the injury if a fracture also exists. Therefore it is strongly advised that the existence and severity of a fracture be determined before performing stress radiographic procedures. Such stress procedures should always be done in the presence of a physician. Some physicians find it helpful to have such procedures done with the aid of anesthesia; local, regional, or general anesthesia can be used to permit a joint to be stressed for radiographic evaluation. If stress procedures are being performed, there may be some value in doing bilateral comparison studies.

When a patient with a possible joint injury, especially a possible dislocation, is being moved, it is important that both the joint and corresponding limb be well supported. Failure to do so may result in further injury. Patients with a possible upper limb dislocation (i.e., shoulder, elbow, wrist) or other possible upper limb joint injury may be able to support the injured upper limb with the opposite arm. Patients with a possible lower limb dislocation (i.e., hip, knee, ankle) should under no circumstances be allowed to move themselves. When the patient is being moved, direct support of the affected joint and limb should be provided for the patient by another person. The radiographer should be prepared to provide any assistance that may be required while the patient is being moved.

Some patients with possible joint injuries may have a sling or splint on the affected limb at the time of the radiographic examination. In some cases it may be desirable to remove the sling or splint because it will interfere with the examination. Slings and splints should be removed by only the radiographer, not the patient, after having obtained permission of the physician to do so and in the presence of a physician.

Patients with Possible Fractures

Fractures vary widely in severity. The presence or severity of a fracture is not always obvious. Until the full extent of the patient's injury has been determined, for the purpose of prudent patient care, the radiographer should treat the patient as if a fracture exists. Patients should always be questioned about the pain they are feeling before any radiographic procedure is begun. Procedures that necessitate the movement of a possibly fractured bone or the application of pressure on a possibly fractured bone may exacerbate the injury to that bone and surrounding tissues; this movement should always be done with caution. Radiographic procedures must be selected with the possibility of fracture in mind. If the patient seems unable to move or put pressure on the bone in question, the radiographer should consult the physician concerning the radiographs to be produced. No patient should be forced into a radiographic position if it is obviously painful to do so. The physician, in consultation with the radiographer, should be the only person to decide whether the radiographic procedure should be completed based on the condition of the patient.

When a patient with a possible fracture is being moved, it is important that both the fracture and corresponding limb be well supported. Failure to do so may result in further injury. Patients with a possibly fractured arm may be able to support the injured upper limb with the opposite arm. Patients with a possible lower limb fracture, however, may require the direct assistance of another person to support the fractured bone and corresponding limb. Patients with possible vertebral column or pelvic fractures should under no circumstances be allowed to move themselves. The radiographer should be prepared to provide any assistance while the patient is being moved. A patient with a possible vertebral column injury should be moved only under the direct supervision of a physician.

Special Care of Severely Traumatized Patients

Patients who have been severely traumatized may suffer from a variety of injuries, some of which may not be orthopedic. The physician may order radiographic examinations to determine the extent of neurologic, respiratory, or cardiac injury before attempting to determine the extent of orthopedic injury. In these instances it is important for the radiographer to perform all radiographic procedures with the possibility of orthopedic injury in mind. That is, it is important not to move a possibly injured joint or fractured bone without the direct consent of a physician while performing all radiographic procedures.

In the case of a severely traumatized patient the atypical orthopedic radiographic procedures presented here may not be applicable or advisable, at least not initially. Usually, in cases of severe trauma the radiographer is extremely limited in the extent of radiographic examinations that can be performed. This is especially true in the case of orthopedic examinations. Often, patients with orthopedic trauma will also have neurologic, respiratory, or cardiac trauma that is of higher priority to immediately assess and treat. In these cases only the simplest of orthopedic radiographic examinations may be performed. The atypical orthopedic radiographic procedures presented here may, in some cases of severe trauma, be used only if the patient is reasonably able to cooperate. In any case, the physician should always make the final determination of the scope and extent of any radiographic procedure to be performed.

EXPOSURE FACTORS IN ORTHOPEDIC RADIOGRAPHY

In orthopedic radiography special care must be taken in the selection of various exposure factors and imaging parameters to ensure that the best radiograph possible is produced. Such care will increase the utility of the procedures presented here, thereby increasing their value. The ideal is to achieve radiographs that demonstrate bone trabeculation and surrounding soft tissues. Although it is beyond the scope of this book to present a thorough discussion of radiographic exposure, the way in which exposure factors and imaging parameters can be manipulated to enhance the value of orthopedic radiography will be discussed.

Selecting a Film-Screen Combination

A variety of radiographic films and intensifying screens are available for use in orthopedic radiography. The speed of the film and the speed of the intensifying screens determine the speed of the combined film-screen system. As a rule, the faster a film-screen system is, the poorer the recorded detail (sharpness) and resolution of the radiographs produced by this system will be. Recorded detail refers to the ability to radiographically produce images with sharp edges; resolution refers to the ability to radiographically record very small structures or features. Recorded detail and resolution are perhaps more important in orthopedic radiography than in other areas of radiography because of the characteristics of the anatomy being visualized. Subtle fractures and changes in bone trabeculae may be missed on radiographs produced with fast film-screen combinations. Therefore it is desirable to select an imaging system that produces a high degree of recorded detail and resolution. On the other hand, it is also desirable to select an imaging system that does not require significantly high exposure factors. As a rule, faster film-screen systems require lower exposure factors to produce the desired amount of film blackening. The use of lower exposure factors has the advantages of decreasing patient exposure to radiation and decreasing wear and tear on radiographic equipment. Therefore it is necessary to choose a system or systems that produce a good compromise between image quality and patient exposure.

Film-screen systems that have a speed rating of 100 or less are most appropriate for radiographic imaging of the limbs and are marketed as "detail" or "extremity" systems. A somewhat faster system is desirable for thicker body parts, such as the vertebral column or pelvis, to eliminate the necessity of unreasonably high exposure factors. A relatively recent innovation in radiographic film manufacturing is of probable benefit to orthopedic radiography. Tabular grain, or T-grain technology film, produces improved recorded detail and resolution when compared with conventional technology film but uses less silver. Another less recent innovation in screen technology is also of potential benefit to orthopedic radiography. Rare earth phosphor screens are faster than comparable calcium tungstate screens, but produce recorded detail and resolution comparable with that produced by calcium tungstate. One can, therefore, use lower exposure factors with rare earth screens and not sacrifice image quality. Radiographic film technical sales representatives can further assist in selecting an imaging system or systems for a facility's particular needs.

Selecting kVp and mAs

When producing any radiograph it is necessary to select the proper exposure factors that produce the desired levels of radiographic density (film blackening) and radiographic contrast (differences in the various shades of gray found on a radiograph). The peak kilovoltage (kVp) used should be sufficient to penetrate the anatomic part, but not so intense that radiographic contrast is diminished. In general, as kVp increases, the penetrating ability of the primary x-ray beam increases but radiographic contrast decreases. Thicker anatomic parts require greater kVp because they are more difficult to penetrate. Exceptions to this rule are structures that comprise the anterior bony thorax, such as the sternum and sternoclavicular (SC) joints. The lungs, which are in close proximity to these structures, are easy to penetrate. Therefore anatomic part thickness plays less of a role in determining proper kVp levels for the SC joints and sternum.

The amount of milliampere seconds (mAs) used should be sufficient to produce the desired level of radiographic density. As a rule, as mAs increases, radiographic density increases proportionately. In most cases it is beneficial to use as short an exposure time as possible to eliminate the imaging of patient motion. In these cases a higher mA value should be used to produce a particular mAs value. In some cases a longer-than-usual exposure time, perhaps seconds, is beneficial to image patient motion of surrounding anatomic structures so that the structure of interest is better visualized. Two such procedures of the sternum are presented in Chapter 4. Lower mA stations usually allow an exposure to be made by using a small focal spot; this has the advantage of increased recorded detail and resolution. To achieve the very shortest exposure time possible, however, a higher mA station must be used. A compromise can usually be struck when radiographing very small anatomic parts by allowing low mA stations and small focal spot sizes to be used with relatively short exposure times.

If either factor, kVp or mAs, is properly set for a particular anatomic part while the other factor is not, an unsatisfactory radiograph will be produced. The combination of kVp and mAs must be such that a properly exposed radiograph is produced. When establishing new exposure factors for a new radiographic installation, a recently calibrated radiographic unit, or a different film-screen system, it is helpful to use a radiographic phantom to establish some baseline exposure factors. Such phantoms can be prohibitively expensive but can usually be found in radiographer training programs and perhaps borrowed for a short period for such use. A radiographic film technical sales representative probably can assist in establishing some baseline exposure factors for selected anatomic parts.

Regulating Focal-Film Distance and Object-Film Distance

Focal-film distance (FFD), or source-image distance (SID), refers to the distance between the x-ray tube focal spot and the radiographic film. Object-film distance (OFD), or object-image distance (OID), refers to the distance between the object being radiographed and the radiographic film. These geometric relationships are important in producing radiographs with desired levels of recorded detail. Most orthopedic radiography is performed using an FFD (SID) of 1 meter (40 inches), which generally produces good image quality. If desired, a decreased FFD (SID) can be used to produce a magnified radiographic image. As a rule, as FFD (SID) decreases, magnification of the radiographic image increases. Fodor and Malott[1] indicate that magnification radiography may be of value in demonstrating erosive arthropathies, metabolic bone diseases, small fractures, and early osteonecrosis that may not otherwise be demonstrated. However, as FFD (SID) decreases, recorded detail also decreases. Therefore, when magnification radiography is performed, FFD (SID) should be decreased in moderation to minimize the decrease in the radiograph's recorded detail.

Object-film distance is virtually zero for tabletop radiography or may be as much as 3 or 4 inches (8 to 11 cm) when a film holder or Bucky device is used. These OFDs (OIDs) generally produce good image quality. If desired, an increased OFD (OID) can be used to produce a magnified radiographic image. As a rule, as OFD (OID) increases, magnification of the radiographic image increases. However, as OFD (OID) increases, recorded detail decreases. Therefore, when magnification radiography is performed, OFD (OID) should be increased in moderation to minimize the decrease in the radiograph's recorded detail.

In orthopedic radiography a small focal spot size should be used whenever possible to maximize recorded detail and resolution. This is especially true for magnification procedures in which recorded detail will be diminished.

Controlling Beam Alignment

The proper alignment of the central ray (CR) to the anatomic part being radiographed, the film, and the grid is important. In all cases the CR should be directed to either enter or exit at the specific anatomic part of interest, depending on patient positioning. This will ensure that radiographic distortion from beam divergence is kept at a minimum. For example, if an AP projection of an SC joint is to be produced, the CR should be directed to *enter* at that joint. If, however, a PA projection of an SC joint is to be produced, the CR should be directed to *exit* at that joint. Simply stated, the CR should always pass directly through the anatomic structure of interest.

The CR should always be directed to the center of the film, or the portion thereof, being used. This will ensure that the exposure is properly centered on the radiograph. The CR should only be angled against the longitudinal axis of the grid being used and should always be directed to enter the center of the grid. This will ensure that grid cutoff does not occur as a result of beam divergence or grid focus. It will also ensure that the CR is being directed to the center of the film. In all cases each radiographic procedure presented here indicates the proper angle, if any, of the CR to the part, film, and grid. The proper entrance or exit point of the CR for each radiographic procedure is also presented here. These relationships are also visually demonstrated for the benefit of the reader.

Selecting and Using a Grid

Grids are generally used in radiographing body parts that are thicker than 9 cm (3½ inches). The grid absorbs some scatter radiation that would otherwise decrease radiographic contrast. Grids are used as part of a Bucky device or are available separately as a wafer grid, as a tunnel grid, or as a grid that is permanently bonded to a cassette. A wide variety of grids are available; they vary in terms of grid ratio, grid pattern, and grid focus. In orthopedic radiography, if a practitioner were to use only a single grid for all procedures requiring a grid, the best compromise among all these factors would be a midratio grid (6:1–10:1), which has a linear pattern as opposed to a crossed pattern, is focused as opposed to parallel, and accommodates a 1-meter (40-inch) FFD (SID) in its focal range. Such a grid produces a moderate amount of contrast improvement, is relatively easy for the radiographer to use, and requires only moderate increases in the exposure factors necessary to produce a diagnostic radiograph.

Anatomic parts less than 9 cm (3½ inches) thick do not require the use of a grid because they produce very little scatter radiation. Radiography of such parts is best done with the part in direct contact with the film cassette. Anatomic parts that measure exactly 9 cm (3½ inches) in thickness may be radiographed with or without the use of a grid. Satisfactory radiographs of some body parts that measure very close to 9 cm (3½ inches), such as the typical adult knee, can be made with or without a grid, depending on the personal preference of the radiographer or physician.

Portable Orthopedic Radiography

Portable orthopedic radiography represents somewhat more of a challenge than orthopedic radiography done in a regular radiographic room. If the standard radiographic room is considered a "controlled" environment, the environment in which portable radiography takes place can then be described as "uncontrolled." That is, the parameters of kVp, mAs, FFD (SID), and OFD (OID) used and controlled in the radiographic room may now be somewhat more restricted.

Many portable radiographic units do not allow the wide range of technical factor selection that fixed-installation units allow. Portable units are usually more restrictive in terms of the total range of kVp and mAs that can be used. With many portable units, exposure time cannot be controlled as a separate factor; instead, mAs is controlled as a single factor that combines both mA and exposure time. Such units, therefore, do not allow one to necessarily use short or long exposure times selectively.

The FFD (SID) and OFD (OID) used in portable radiography may vary from what are normally used in the radiographic room, but they may be standardized. Variation could be a result of the physical size of the room where the patient is radiographed, patient position during the examination, or physical limitations of the portable unit. Standardization may be accomplished by *always:* placing the portable unit in the same position with respect to the bed or cart; performing the examination with the bed or cart at a standard distance from the floor; elevating the back of the bed or cart, if necessary, to the same upright angle; raising the tube to the same height; and producing the same degree of tube angle, if necessary, for each similar type of examination. Technical factors for each similar type of examination should also be standardized. This can be done by recording the factors used for a particular examination, in addition to patient or part thickness, and using those same factors in similar situations.

It is also important to be especially careful of the alignment of the CR to the patient, film, and grid during portable radiography. Alignment is fairly easy to achieve in the radiographic room, but is somewhat more difficult when a portable unit is used. Before any exposure is made, it is necessary to evaluate the relationship of the x-ray tube, patient, film, and grid to one another. The relationships should be exactly the same whether the examination is performed in the radiographic room or with a portable unit.

Adjusting for Casts and Splints

Frequently in orthopedic radiography, radiographs are produced with the anatomic part of interest in a cast or splint. Dry plaster casts require that the mAs be increased by at least 2 times the normal mAs required for the part. If the part is large, such as a femur, or if a large amount of plaster is present, mAs may need to be increased by 3 times the normal mAs required for the part. Wet plaster casts require that the mAs be increased by at least 3 times the normal mAs required for the part. If the part is large or a large amount of plaster was used, mAs may need to be increased by 4 times the normal mAs required for the part. Fiberglass casts generally require no increase in exposure factors. Detail or extremity-speed intensifying screens should not be used for radiographing parts in casts. Instead, a higher speed system should be used to avoid excessive imaging of the cast itself.

Splints produce less of a problem with necessary exposure. Air (inflatable), plastic, and fiberglass splints do not require any increase in exposure factors. Wood and aluminum splints may require that exposure factors be increased. If two pieces of wood are bound to the sides of a lower leg, for example, no increase in exposure factors is necessary for an AP projection because the splint does not interfere with the radiographic image. In the same scenario, however, if a lateral radiograph is taken, the splint interferes with the radiographic imaging of the part and necessitates an increase in exposure factors. An increase of 5 kVp or 50% in mAs over normal should produce a properly exposed radiograph when a wood or aluminum splint is in the path of the primary or transmitted x-ray beam.

Splints may produce radiographic artifacts. It may, therefore, be desirable to remove the splint before the radiographic procedure is performed. It is essential that a splint be removed only with permission of a physician and in the presence of a physician. Extra care should be taken to provide proper support for the joint and/or limb from which a splint is removed.

CHAPTER 1 • REFERENCE

1. Fodor J, Malott JC: Magnification radiography, *Radiol Technol* 58:313, 1987.

CHAPTER
2
The Upper Limb

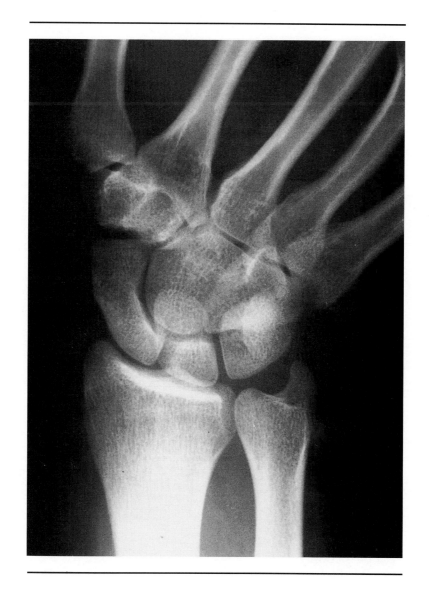

❖ First Digit

AP STRESS PROJECTIONS

Pathology Demonstrated. Instability of the metacarpophalangeal joint of the first digit (thumb).

Often, routine methods of demonstrating the first digit do not demonstrate ligamentous injuries. Instability of the metacarpophalangeal joint is demonstrated radiographically as an abnormal increase in joint mobility. O'Brien[10] indicates that stability of the metacarpophalangeal joint can be assessed by stressing the first digit laterally (Figure 2-1) and medially (Figure 2-2). Patients who are experiencing a substantial amount of pain should not be examined in this manner without anesthesia.

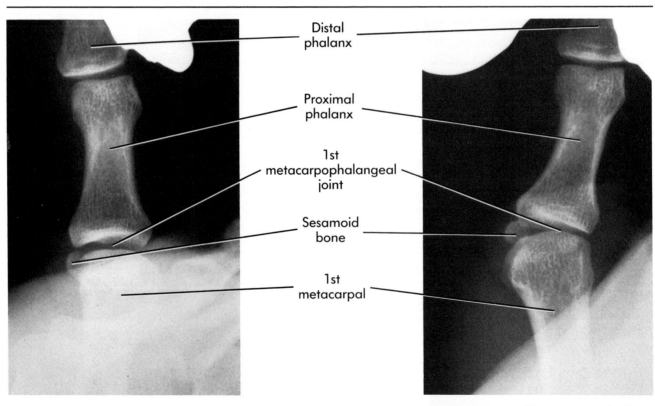

Distal phalanx

Proximal phalanx

1st metacarpophalangeal joint

Sesamoid bone

1st metacarpal

FIGURE 2-1 AP stress projection.

FIGURE 2-2 AP stress projection.

Patient Position. The patient should be seated with the affected hand positioned in maximum internal rotation, placing the radial surface of the hand on the cassette, which is placed on the radiographic tabletop.

Part Position. Two AP projections of the first digit should be produced. For the first exposure the first digit should be stressed laterally (Figure 2-3). For the second exposure the first digit should be stressed medially (Figure 2-4). Be certain that the person providing the stress wears lead gloves and a lead apron during both exposures.

Central Ray. The central ray should be directed perpendicular to the film to enter at the metacarpophalangeal joint.

Radiograph Evaluation. The metacarpophalangeal joint of the first digit should be demonstrated without superimposition of the hand and without rotation.

The first digit should be stressed both laterally and medially.

The metacarpophalangeal joint and the bony trabeculae should be well visualized.

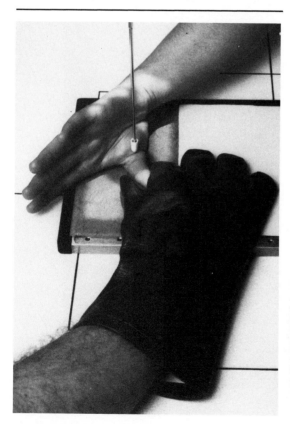

FIGURE 2-3   AP stress projection.

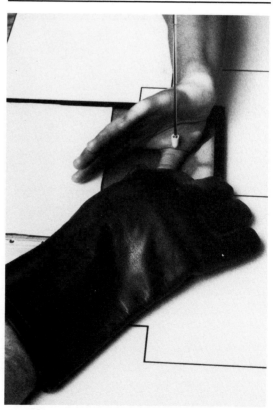

FIGURE 2-4   AP stress projection.

PA STRESS PROJECTION

Pathology Demonstrated. Instability of the interphalangeal joint of the first digit (thumb).

Instability of the interphalangeal joint is demonstrated radiographically by an abnormal increase in joint mobility. Stability of the interphalangeal joint can be assessed by pinching the first digit with the second digit of the same hand (Figure 2-5). This technique should not be used with patients who are experiencing a substantial amount of pain. The method is, however, valuable for patients who are able to cooperate.

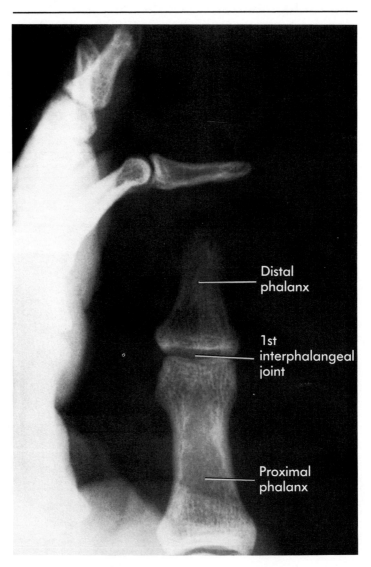

Distal phalanx

1st interphalangeal joint

Proximal phalanx

FIGURE 2-5   PA stress projection.

Patient Position. The patient should be seated with the ulnar surface of the affected hand on the cassette, which is placed on the radiographic tabletop.

Part Position. The affected first digit should be positioned as for a PA projection. Have the patient place stress on the distal phalanx of the first digit by using the second digit to push longitudinally (Figure 2-6).

Central Ray. The central ray should be directed perpendicular to the film to enter at the interphalangeal joint.

Radiograph Evaluation. The first digit should be demonstrated without rotation.

The first digit should not be flexed at the interphalangeal joint, but instead should be extended to allow for accurate evaluation of the joint space.

The interphalangeal joint and bony trabeculae should be well visualized.

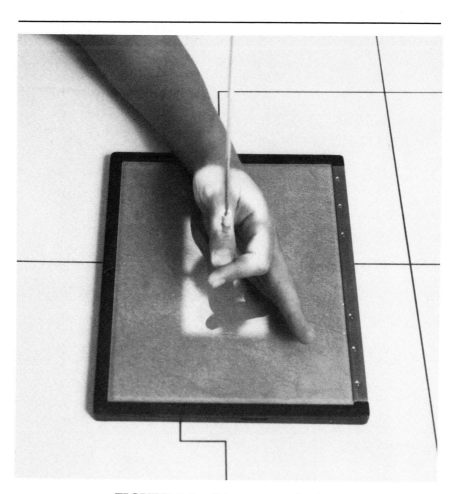

FIGURE 2-6   PA stress projection.

HAND

❖ Hand

AP PROJECTION

Pathology Demonstrated. Small detached fracture fragments at the bases of the metacarpals.

The routine PA projection of the hand does not adequately demonstrate small detached fragments that may be present at the bases of the metacarpals as a result of a fracture injury to the hand. Murless[9] indicates that an AP projection (Figure 2-7) can be used to demonstrate the bases of the metacarpals more successfully.

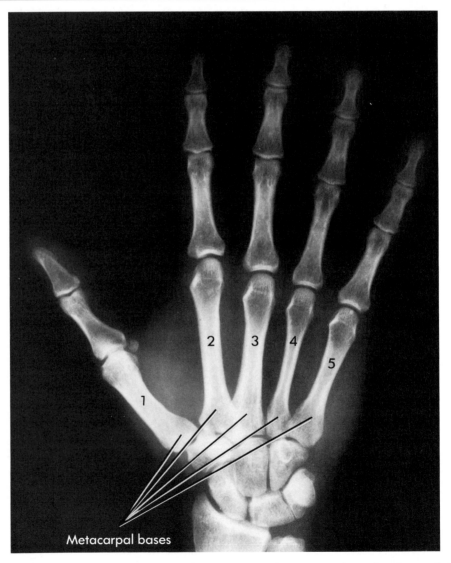

FIGURE 2-7 AP projection. The metacarpals are numbered 1 through 5.

Patient Position. The patient should be seated with the affected hand on the cassette, which is placed on the radiographic tabletop.

Part Position. The hand should be positioned with the dorsal surface in contact with the cassette. The digits should be slightly spread and extended (Figure 2-8).

Central Ray. The central ray should be directed perpendicular to the film to enter at the midmetacarpal region.

Radiograph Evaluation. The hand should be demonstrated without rotation.

The digits should be slightly spread and extended.

The bases of the metacarpals should be adequately penetrated, and the bony trabeculae of the entire hand should be well visualized.

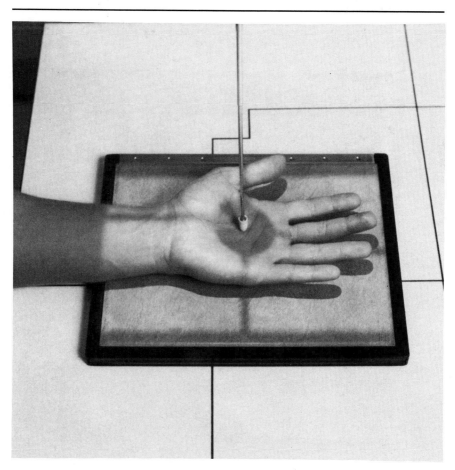

FIGURE 2-8   AP projection.

AP OBLIQUE (PALMODORSAL) POSITION

Pathology Demonstrated. Small detached fracture fragments at the bases of the metacarpals.

Small detached fracture fragments of the hand may not be demonstrated with routine methods. Bora and Didzian[2] indicate that the AP oblique position of the hand (Figure 2-9) is valuable for assessing the bases of the metacarpals for this purpose.

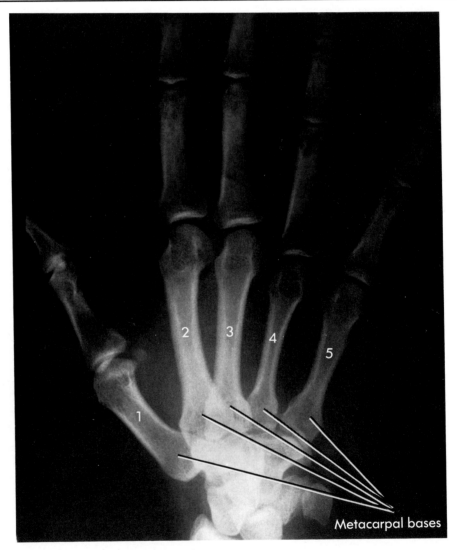

FIGURE 2-9   AP oblique (palmodorsal) position. The metacarpals are numbered 1 through 5.

Patient Position. The patient should be seated with the affected hand on the cassette, which is placed on the radiographic tabletop.

Part Position. The hand should be positioned as for an AP projection with the dorsal surface in contact with the cassette. The hand should then be rotated internally 30 degrees with the digits slightly spread and extended (Figure 2-10).

Central Ray. The central ray should be directed perpendicular to the film to enter at the midpoint of the midmetacarpal region.

Radiograph Evaluation. The bases of the metacarpals should be demonstrated.

The digits should be slightly spread and extended.

The bases of the metacarpals should be adequately penetrated and the bony trabeculae well visualized.

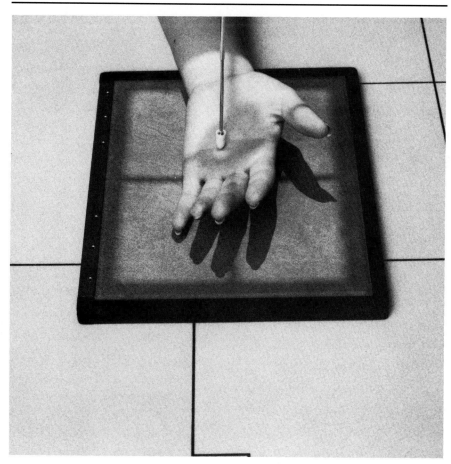

FIGURE 2-10 AP oblique (palmodorsal) position.

HAND

AP (PALMODORSAL) AND PA (DORSOPALMAR) OBLIQUE POSITIONS

Pathology Demonstrated. Angulation of metacarpal fractures.

True lateral positions or standard oblique positions of the hand do not often demonstrate the angulation of metacarpal fractures. Green and Rowland[5] indicate that two slightly oblique positions in both directions from the lateral (Figures 2-11 and 2-12) are useful for this purpose.

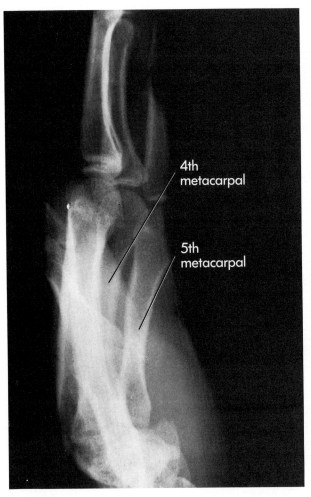

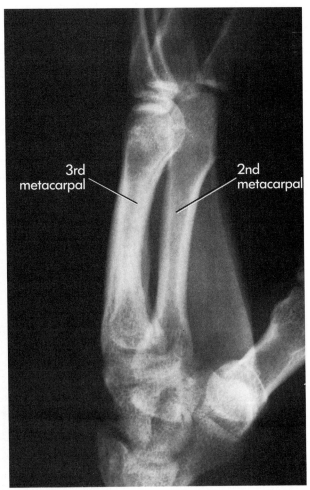

FIGURE 2-11   AP oblique (palmodorsal) position.

FIGURE 2-12   PA oblique (dorsopalmar) position.

Patient Position. The patient should be seated with the ulnar surface of the affected hand on the cassette, which is placed on the radiographic tabletop.

Part Position. Two different oblique positions should be achieved. To demonstrate the fourth and fifth metacarpals the hand should be supinated 10 degrees from the lateral position (palmodorsal oblique) with the second through fourth digits extended and in contact with one another (Figure 2-13). To demonstrate the second and third metacarpals the hand should be pronated 10 degrees from the lateral position (dorsopalmar oblique) with the second through fourth digits extended and in contact with one another (Figure 2-14). For both positions the first digit (thumb) should be extended and abducted to prevent superimposition over the metacarpals of interest.

Central Ray. The central ray should be directed perpendicular to the film to enter at the midmetacarpal region.

Radiograph Evaluation. The fourth and fifth metacarpals should be demonstrated with the palmodorsal (supination) oblique.

The second and third metacarpals should be demonstrated with the dorsopalmar (pronation) oblique.

The first digit should not superimpose the metacarpals of interest for either position.

The bony trabeculae of the respective metacarpals should be well visualized.

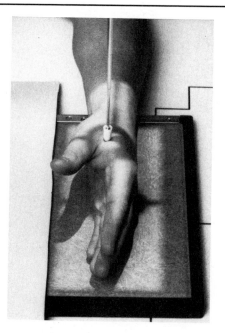

FIGURE 2-13 AP oblique (palmodorsal) position.

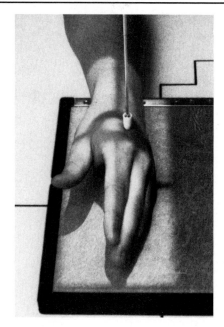

FIGURE 2-14 PA oblique (dorsopalmar) position.

HAND

AP AXIAL POSITION: 20-DEGREE BREWERTON METHOD

Pathology Demonstrated. Erosion of the metacarpal heads and bases of the phalanges.

Bony erosion of the metacarpal heads and bases of the phalanges as a result of rheumatoid arthritis is not well visualized with routine methods. Stoker and Horsfield[11] indicate that this method is useful for demonstrating the second through fifth metacarpal heads and the bases of the second through fifth phalanges for this purpose (Figure 2-15).

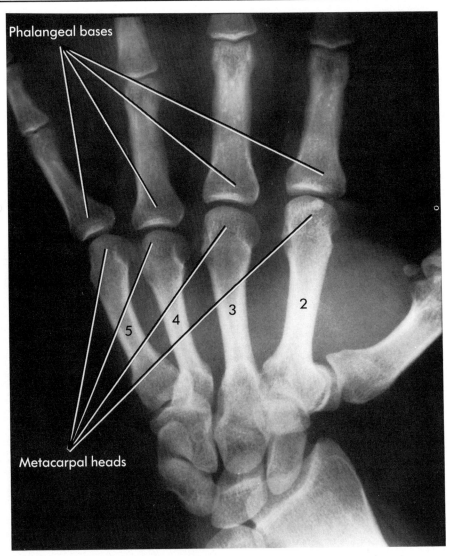

FIGURE 2-15   AP axial position: 20-degree Brewerton Method. The metacarpals are numbered 2 through 5.

Patient Position. The patient should be standing beside the radiographic table with the dorsal surface of the hand on the cassette, which is placed on the radiographic tabletop.

Part Position. The digits should be kept flat on the cassette with the metacarpophalangeal joints flexed away from the cassette at a 45-degree angle. There should be no flexion of the wrist joint, and the digits should be slightly spread and extended (Figure 2-16). An angle sponge positioned under the metacarpals and wrist assists the patient in maintaining this position.

Central Ray. The central ray should be angled laterally 20 degrees and directed to enter at the third metacarpophalangeal joint.

Radiograph Evaluation. The metacarpal heads, metacarpophalangeal joints, and the bases of the phalanges should be demonstrated.

The wrist should not be flexed.

The digits should be somewhat spread and extended.

The bony trabeculae of the metacarpal heads and bases of the phalanges should be well visualized.

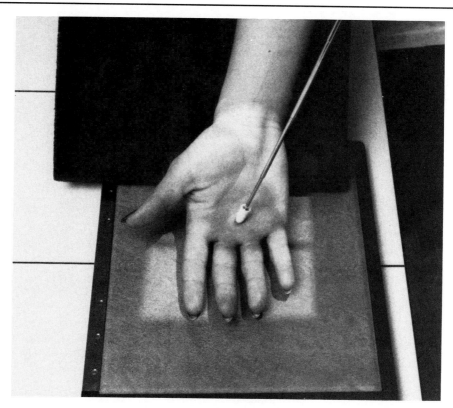

FIGURE 2-16   AP axial position: 20-degree Brewerton Method.

AP AXIAL POSITION: 30-DEGREE BREWERTON METHOD

Pathology Demonstrated. Occult fractures of the metacarpal bases.

Fractures of the metacarpal bases may be difficult to visualize with routine methods. Kaye and Lister[6] indicate that this method is useful for demonstrating the metacarpal bases for this purpose (Figure 2-17).

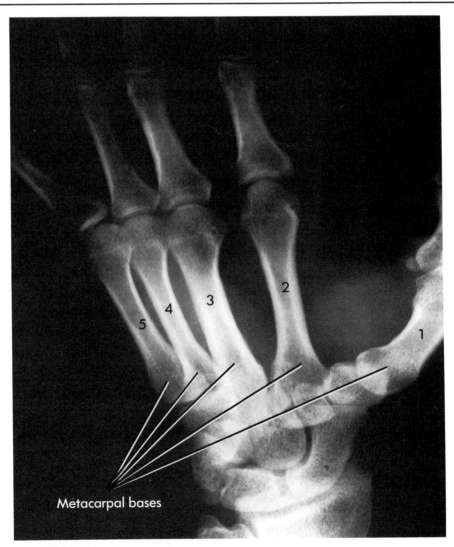

FIGURE 2-17   AP axial position: 30-degree Brewerton Method. The metacarpals are numbered 1 through 5.

Patient Position. The patient should be seated beside the radiographic table with the dorsal surface of the affected hand on the cassette, which is placed on the radiographic tabletop.

Part Position. The digits should be kept flat on the cassette with the metacarpophalangeal joints flexed away from the cassette 45 degrees and the wrist dorsiflexed 45 degrees. The digits should be extended and somewhat spread (Figure 2-18).

Central Ray. The central ray should be angled laterally 30 degrees and directed to enter at the base of the third metacarpal.

Radiograph Evaluation. The metacarpal bases should be well demonstrated.
   The digits should be extended and spread.
   The bony trabeculae of the bases of the metacarpals should be well visualized.

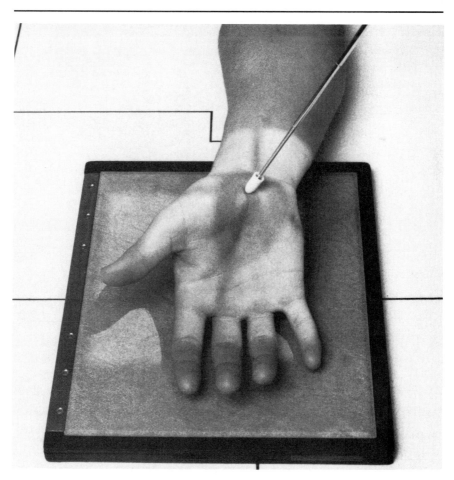

FIGURE 2-18   AP axial position: 30-degree Brewerton Method.

❖ Wrist

AP CARPAL COMPRESSION PROJECTION

Pathology Demonstrated. Subluxation of the scaphoid (navicular) and lunate.

Widening of the scapholunate articulation as a result of wrist trauma is often not visualized with routine wrist radiography. Dobyns and others[4] indicate that AP compression projections of the wrist are useful for this purpose (Figures 2-19 and 2-20). Patients who are experiencing a substantial amount of pain should not be examined in this manner. This method is, however, valuable for those patients who are able to cooperate.

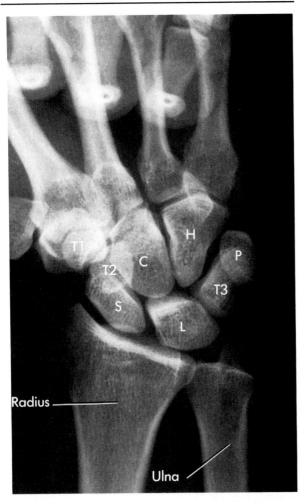

FIGURE 2-19 AP carpal compression projection. *T1*, trapezium; *T2*, trapezoid; *C*, capitate; *H*, hamate; *P*, pisiform; *T3*, triquetrum; *L*, lunate; *S*, scaphoid.

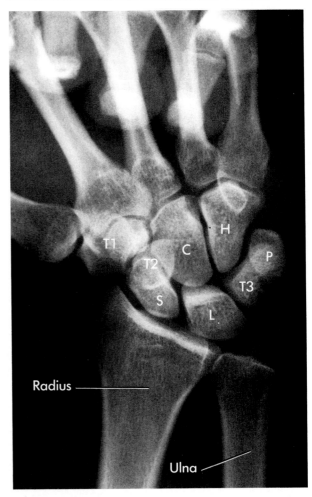

FIGURE 2-20 AP carpal compression projection. *T1*, trapezium; *T2*, trapezoid; *C*, capitate; *H*, hamate; *P*, pisiform; *T3*, triquetrum; *L*, lunate; *S*, scaphoid.

Patient Position. The patient should be seated with the dorsal surface of the affected wrist on the cassette, which is placed on the radiographic tabletop.

Part Position. Either or both compression methods may be of value. For the first method the wrist is positioned for an AP projection with the patient forming a tight fist (Figure 2-21). For the second method the wrist is again positioned for an AP projection with the patient forming a tight fist; additional compression is provided by another person placing his or her hand against the fist and pushing longitudinally (Figure 2-22). Be certain that the person providing the compression wears lead gloves and a lead apron during compression exposures.

Central Ray. For both AP projections the central ray should be directed perpendicular to enter at the midcarpal region.

Radiograph Evaluation. The bony trabeculae of the scaphoid and lunate should be well visualized.

The space between the scaphoid and lunate should be well visualized.

Compression should be provided to demonstrate possible widening of the articulation between the scaphoid and lunate.

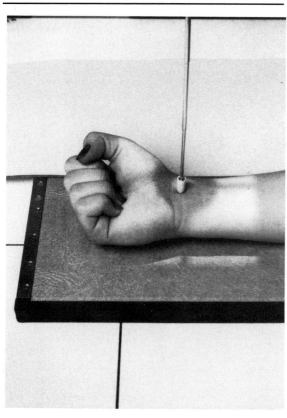

FIGURE 2-21 AP carpal compression projection.

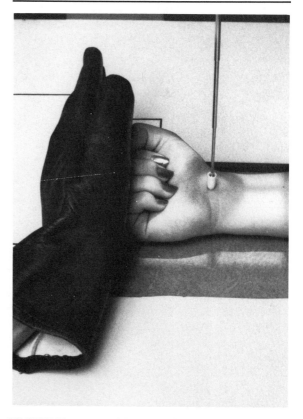

FIGURE 2-22 AP carpal compression projection.

PA 10-DEGREE AXIAL POSITION

Pathology Demonstrated. Subluxation of the scaphoid (navicular) and lunate.

Another method for demonstrating widening of the space between the scaphoid and lunate also exists. Kindynis and others[7] indicate that a PA axial position of the wrist is useful for this purpose (Figure 2-23).

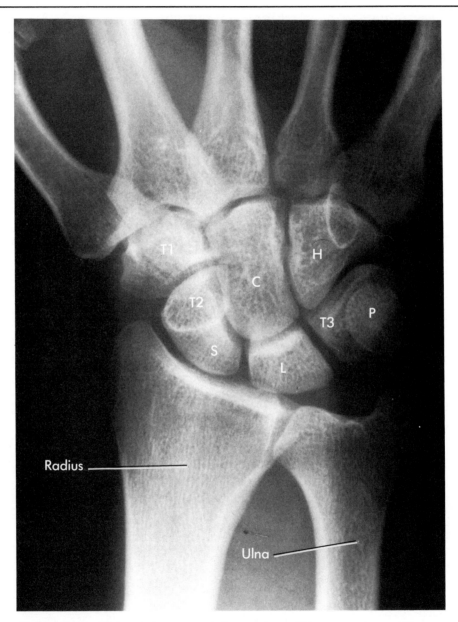

FIGURE 2-23 PA 10-degree axial position. *T1*, trapezium; *T2*, trapezoid; *C*, capitate; *H*, hamate; *P*, pisiform; *T3*, triquetrum; *L*, lunate; *S*, scaphoid.

Patient Position. The patient should be seated with the affected wrist placed on the cassette, which is placed on the radiographic tabletop as for a PA projection.

Part Position. With the wrist positioned as for a PA projection the digits should be flexed and placed in contact with the cassette to bring the carpals closer to the film (Figure 2-24).

Central Ray. The central ray should be angled 10 degrees medially and directed to enter at the midcarpal region.

Radiograph Evaluation. The bony trabeculae of the scaphoid and lunate should be well visualized.

The space between the scaphoid and lunate should be well visualized.

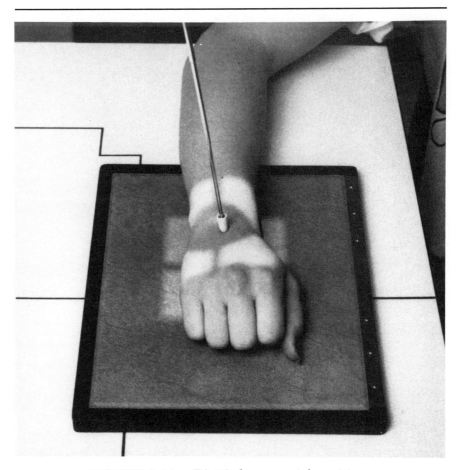

FIGURE 2-24　PA 10-degree axial position.

AP AND PA RADIAL FLEXION OBLIQUE POSITIONS

Pathology Demonstrated. Scaphoid (navicular) fracture.

Fractures of the scaphoid are frequently difficult to demonstrate with routine methods unless separation of fracture fragments exists. Stoker and Horsfield[11] indicate that an AP radial flexion oblique position (Figure 2-25) and a PA radial flexion oblique position (Figure 2-26) are useful for this purpose regardless of the presence of separated bony fragments.

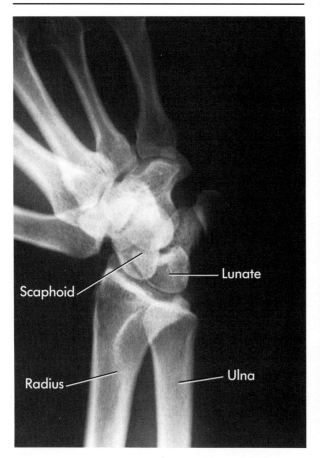

FIGURE 2-25   AP radial flexion oblique position.

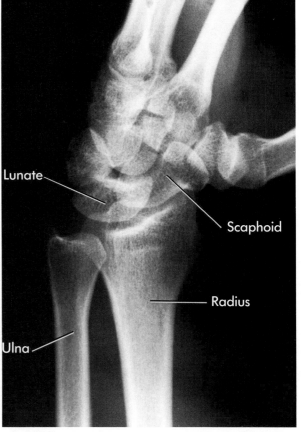

FIGURE 2-26   PA radial flexion oblique position.

Patient Position. The patient should be seated with the dorsal surface of the affected wrist on the cassette, which is placed on the radiographic tabletop.

Part Position. Two radial flexion positions should be achieved. For the first position the wrist should be rotated 30 degrees from the AP with the wrist and hand resting on the ulnar surface. The wrist should then be flexed in maximum radial flexion (Figure 2-27). For the second position the wrist should initially be positioned as for a PA projection. The wrist should be rotated 30 degrees from the PA with the wrist and hand resting on the ulnar surface. The wrist should then be flexed in maximum radial flexion (Figure 2-28). The digits should be extended for each position.

Central Ray. The central ray should be directed perpendicular to the film to enter at the midcarpal region.

Radiograph Evaluation. The scaphoid should be demonstrated in both positions.
    The wrist should be demonstrated in radial flexion for both positions.
    The bony trabeculae of the scaphoid should be well visualized.

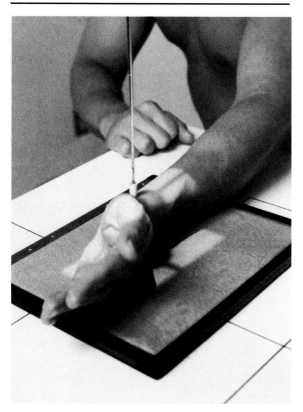

FIGURE 2-27 AP radial flexion oblique position.

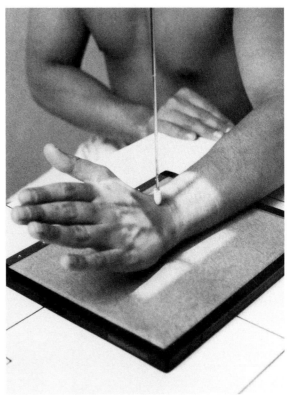

FIGURE 2-28 PA radial flexion oblique position.

PA AXIAL ULNAR FLEXION POSITION

Pathology Demonstrated. Scaphoid (navicular) fracture.

Because scaphoid fractures are often difficult to demonstrate radiographically, other methods are needed. Bontrager[1] indicates that a PA axial position of the wrist with the wrist in ulnar flexion is useful for this purpose (Figure 2-29).

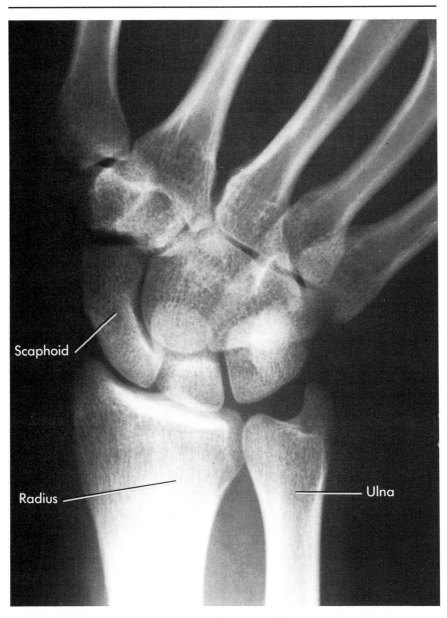

FIGURE 2-29 PA axial ulnar flexion position.

Patient Position. The patient should be seated with the affected wrist on the cassette, which is placed on the radiographic tabletop as for a PA projection.

Part Position. The wrist should be positioned in maximum ulnar flexion with the digits extended (Figure 2-30).

Central Ray. The central ray should be directed at a 20-degree angle longitudinal with the forearm and directed to enter at the midcarpal region.

Radiograph Evaluation. The wrist should be demonstrated in ulnar flexion.
   The scaphoid should be somewhat elongated as a result of the tube angle.
   The bony trabeculae of the scaphoid should be well visualized.

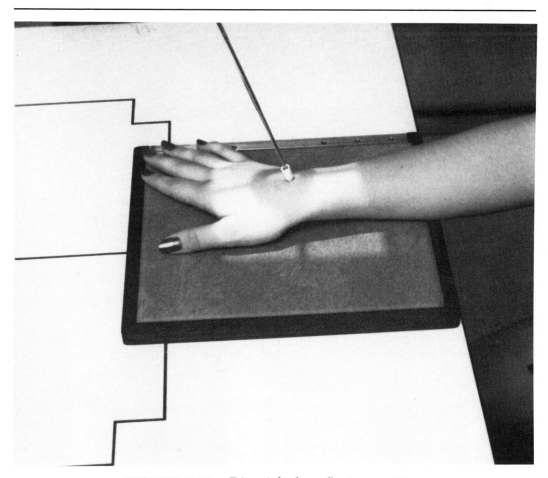

FIGURE 2-30   PA axial ulnar flexion position.

LATERAL FLEXION AND EXTENSION POSITIONS

Pathology Demonstrated. Widening of the wrist joint.

Routine radiography of the wrist joint may not demonstrate widening of the wrist joint, which may be due to fracture, dislocation, or ligamentous injury. McInnes[8] indicates that lateral positions of the wrist in flexion (Figure 2-31) and extension (Figure 2-32) are useful for this purpose.

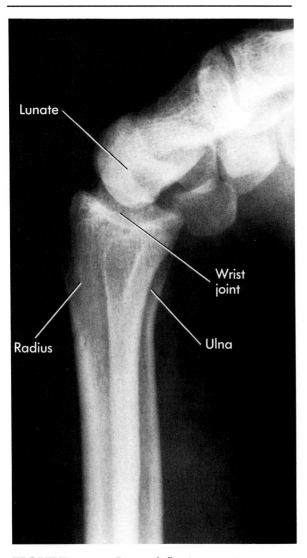

FIGURE 2-31   Lateral flexion position.

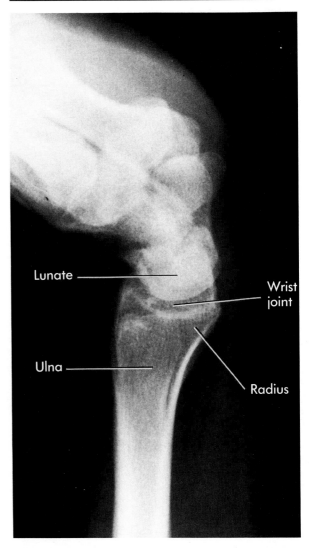

FIGURE 2-32   Lateral extension position.

Patient Position. The patient should be seated with the ulnar surface of the affected wrist on the cassette, which is placed on the radiographic tabletop.

Part Position. Two lateral positions should be achieved. For the first position the wrist should be positioned in maximum flexion (Figure 2-33). For the second position the wrist should be positioned in maximum extension (Figure 2-34).

Central Ray. The central ray should be directed perpendicular to the film to enter at the wrist joint.

Radiograph Evaluation. The wrist should be demonstrated in a true lateral position on both radiographs.

One radiograph should be made with the lateral wrist in flexion and the other radiograph made with the lateral wrist in extension.

The wrist joint and the bony trabeculae of the wrist should be well visualized.

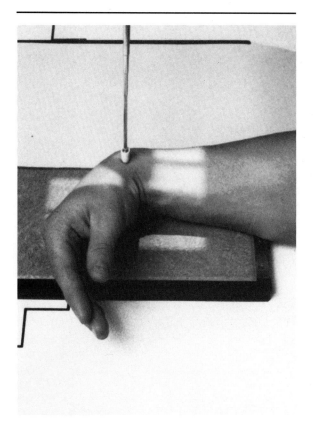

FIGURE 2-33 Lateral flexion position.

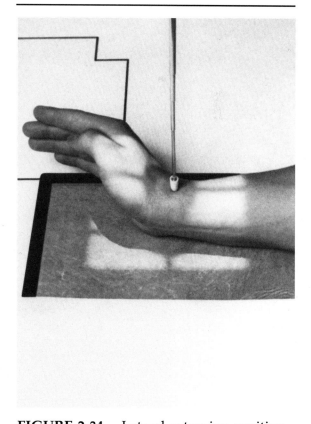

FIGURE 2-34 Lateral extension position.

❖ Elbow

AXIAL LATERAL POSITION

Pathology Demonstrated. Capitulum and radial head fractures.

Routine radiography of the elbow may demonstrate the fat pad sign but no other indication of fracture. DeLee, Green, and Wilkins[3] indicate that the fat pad sign is an area of radiolucency posterior or anterior to the distal humerus as seen in the lateral position and is highly indicative of fracture in this area. If a positive fat pad sign exists on routine radiographs of the elbow but no fracture is apparent, methods other than the routine are needed to demonstrate capitulum and radial head fractures. Stoker and Horsfield[11] indicate that an axial lateral position of the elbow is useful for this purpose (Figure 2-35).

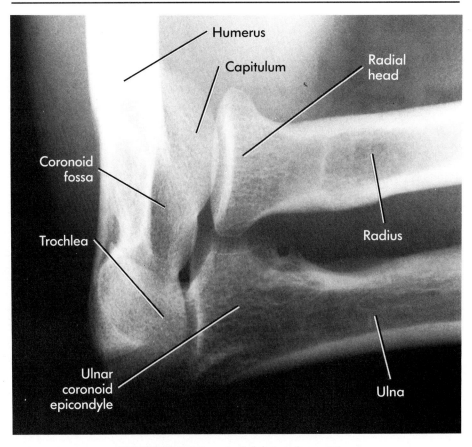

FIGURE 2-35   Axial lateral position.

Patient Position. The patient should be seated with the affected elbow on the cassette, which is placed on the radiographic tabletop.

Part Position. The elbow should be placed in a lateral position with the humerus parallel with the film and tabletop. The wrist and forearm should also be in a lateral position. The elbow should be flexed 90 degrees (Figure 2-36).

Central Ray. The central ray should be angled 45 degrees toward the shoulder along the long axis of the humerus and directed to enter at the elbow joint.

Radiograph Evaluation. The elbow joint should be well visualized.

The capitulum and radial head should appear somewhat elongated.

The bony trabeculae of the capitulum and radial head should be well visualized.

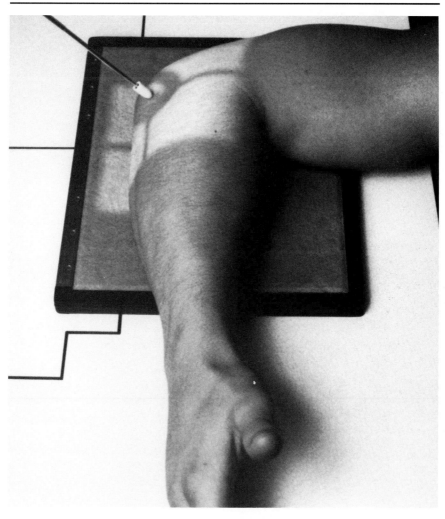

FIGURE 2-36 Axial lateral position.

ELBOW

TRANSABDOMINAL LATERAL POSITION

Pathology Demonstrated. Fracture or dislocation of elbow when arm is immobilized to trunk.

In patients with upper extremity injuries it is frequently difficult to obtain lateral positions of the elbow to demonstrate fracture or dislocation when the arm is immobilized to the trunk. When it is not prudent to remove the immobilization device, other methods must be used.

McInnes[8] suggests that a transabdominal lateral position of the elbow is useful for this purpose (Figure 2-37).

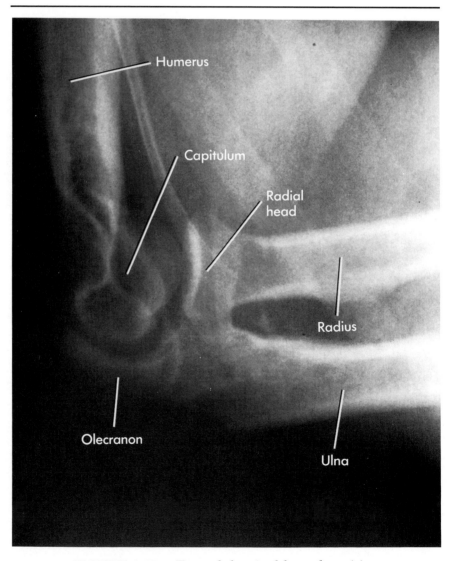

FIGURE 2-37 Transabdominal lateral position.

Patient Position. The patient should be sitting or standing, facing the upright film-holding device which holds the cassette.

Part Position. The patient should be rotated so that the affected elbow is in a lateral position and in contact with the cassette or grid (Figure 2-38). The degree of obliquity at which the patient's trunk should be positioned is dependent on the immobilization that has been applied. The patient should be positioned in a degree of rotation that will not cause superimposition of the vertebral column over the lateral elbow.

Central Ray. The central ray should be directed perpendicular to the film to pass through the lateral elbow joint. This will require that the central ray enter the dorsal surface of the patient at the level of the elbow joint and traverse the abdomen. Swallow and others[12] indicate that if the patient is able to abduct the arm sufficiently to prevent superimposition of the elbow and abdomen, despite the immobilization, the elbow may be radiographed without having the central ray pass through the abdomen.

Radiograph Evaluation. The elbow joint should be demonstrated in a near lateral position.

The vertebral column should not be superimposed over the elbow joint.

The elbow joint and the bony trabeculae of the elbow should be reasonably well visualized.

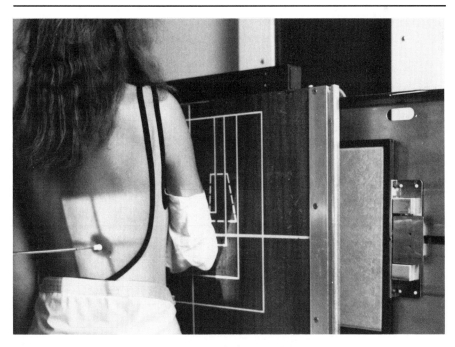

FIGURE 2-38   Transabdominal lateral position.

CHAPTER 2 • REFERENCES

1. Bontrager KL: *Textbook of radiographic positioning and related anatomy,* ed 3, St. Louis, 1993, Mosby–Year Book.
2. Bora FW, Didzian NH: The treatment of injuries to the carpometacarpal joint of the little finger, *J Bone Joint Surg* 56A:1459, 1974.
3. DeLee JC, Green DP, Wilkins KE: *Fractures and dislocations of the elbow.* In Rockwood CA Jr, Green DP, editors: *Fractures in adults,* ed 2, Philadelphia, 1984, JB Lippincott.
4. Dobyns JH and others: Traumatic instability of the wrist, American Academy of Orthopedic Surgeons Instructional Course Lectures 24:182, 1975, St. Louis, Mosby–Year Book.
5. Green DP, Rowland SA: *Fractures and dislocations in the hand.* In Rockwood CA Jr, Green DP, editors: *Fractures in adults,* ed 2, Philadelphia, 1984, JB Lippincott.
6. Kaye JJ, Lister GD: Another use for the Brewerton view, *J Hand Surg* 3:603, 1978.
7. Kindynis P and others: Demonstration of the scapholunate space with radiography, *Radiology* 175:278, 1990.
8. McInnes J: *Clark's positioning in radiography,* ed 9, vol 1, Chicago, 1973, Mosby–Year Book.
9. Murless BC: Fracture-dislocation of the base of the fifth metacarpal bone, *Br J Surg* 31:402, 1943.
10. O'Brien ET: *Fractures of the hand and wrist region.* In Rockwood CA Jr, Wilkins KE, King RE, editors: *Fractures in children,* Philadelphia, 1984, JB Lippincott.
11. Stoker DJ, Horsfield D: *Conventional radiography of the appendicular skeleton.* In Galasko CSB, Isherwood I, editors: *Imaging techniques in orthopaedics,* London, 1989, Springer-Verlag.
12. Swallow RA and others: *Clark's positioning in radiography,* ed 11, Rockville, 1986, Aspen.

The Shoulder Girdle

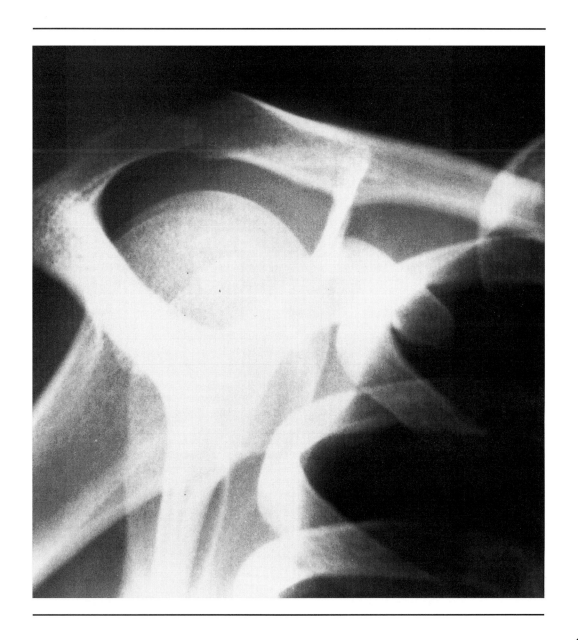

❖ Shoulder

ADDUCTION INFEROSUPERIOR AXIAL POSITION

Pathology Demonstrated. Shoulder dislocation.

Most axillary methods of shoulder radiography require that the patient be able to abduct the humerus from the body so that the shoulder joint can be radiographically demonstrated. In cases of shoulder dislocation, abduction of the humerus is painful and possibly harmful to the patient so other methods must be used. Ciullo, Koniuch, and Teitge[3] have described a method in which the affected arm may remain adducted to demonstrate the relationship of the humeral head to the glenoid cavity (fossa) (Figure 3-1).

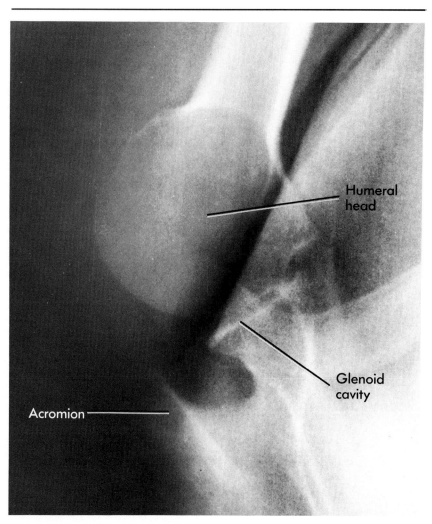

FIGURE 3-1 Adduction inferosuperior axial position.

Patient Position. The patient should be supine on the radiographic table.

Part Position. The affected arm should be elevated off the table with a radiolucent sponge to allow the central ray to pass through the axilla. The humerus should be adducted to the body. The cassette should be placed perpendicular to the tabletop and superior to the shoulder joint.

Central Ray. The horizontal central ray should be directed perpendicular to the film to enter at the axilla (Figure 3-2).

Radiograph Evaluation. The relationship of the humeral head to the glenoid cavity should be demonstrated.

　　The humerus should not be superimposed over the glenoid cavity.
　　The shoulder joint should be well visualized.

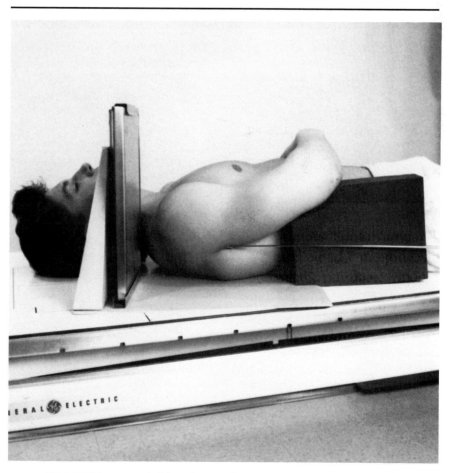

FIGURE 3-2　Adduction inferosuperior axial position.

ADDUCTION SUPEROINFERIOR AXIAL POSITION: VELPEAU METHOD

Pathology Demonstrated. Shoulder dislocation.

Another axillary method that does not require abduction of the humerus from the body is also available for demonstrating the shoulder joint. Bloom and Obata[2] indicate that the Velpeau method is useful for demonstrating the relationship of the humeral head to the glenoid cavity (fossa) when the patient cannot abduct the arm for a normal axillary position (Figure 3-3).

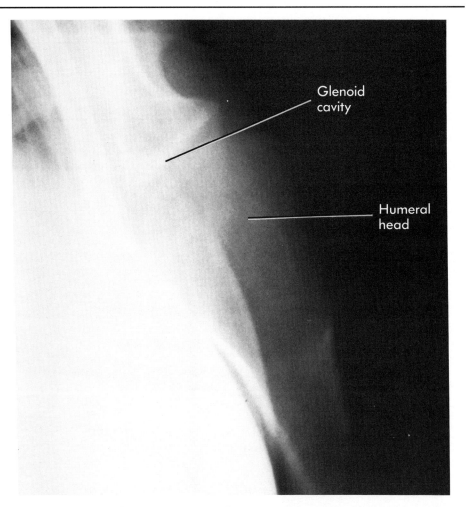

FIGURE 3-3   Adduction superoinferior axial position: Velpeau method.

Patient Position. The patient should be standing with the back against the radiographic table.

Part Position. The humerus should be adducted to the body. If the patient's arm is in a sling or the forearm is otherwise drawn across the trunk, this method can still be used. The patient should lean back over the radiographic table as much as is reasonably possible to prevent superimposition of the shoulder and the trunk (Figure 3-4). The film should be placed below the affected shoulder. To decrease object-film distance (object-image distance), thereby decreasing magnification, a sponge can be used to elevate the film off the radiographic tabletop.

Central Ray. The central ray should be directed perpendicular to the film to enter at the shoulder joint.

Radiograph Evaluation. The relationship of the humeral head to the glenoid cavity should be demonstrated.

The trunk should not be superimposed over the shoulder joint.

Excessive magnification should be avoided by decreasing the distance of the shoulder to the film.

The shoulder joint should be well visualized.

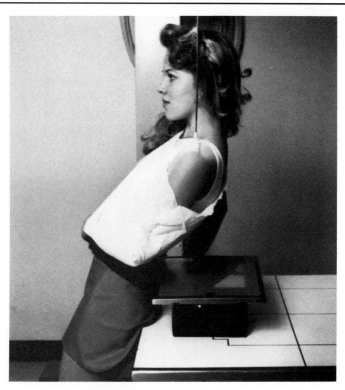

FIGURE 3-4   Adduction superoinferior axial position: Velpeau method.

AP SCAPULAR PLANE POSITION

Pathology Demonstrated. Fracture of the scapula and dislocation of the shoulder.

Routine AP projections of the shoulder and scapula demonstrate the scapula at approximately a 45-degree oblique because of its normal anatomic position within the body. Neer and Rockwood[11] indicate a method that is useful in demonstrating the scapula in a plane parallel with the film (Figure 3-5). This method is also useful for demonstrating shoulder dislocation.

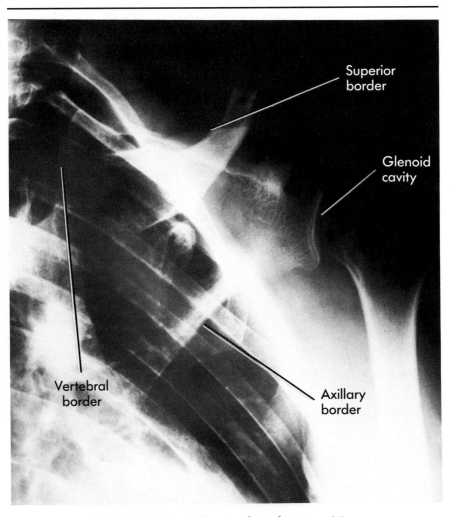

FIGURE 3-5 AP scapular plane position.

Patient Position. The patient should be standing or sitting upright with the back against the upright film-holding device which holds the cassette.

Part Position. To demonstrate the right side the patient should be positioned in a 45-degree RPO. To demonstrate the left side the patient should be positioned in a 45-degree LPO (Figure 3-6). The affected arm should be adducted to the side of the patient.

Central Ray. The central ray should be directed perpendicular to the film to enter 2 inches (5 cm) medial to the glenoid cavity (fossa).

Radiograph Evaluation. The scapula should be demonstrated in an orientation parallel with the film.
　　The glenoid cavity should be demonstrated in profile.
　　The bony trabeculae of the majority of the scapula should be well visualized.

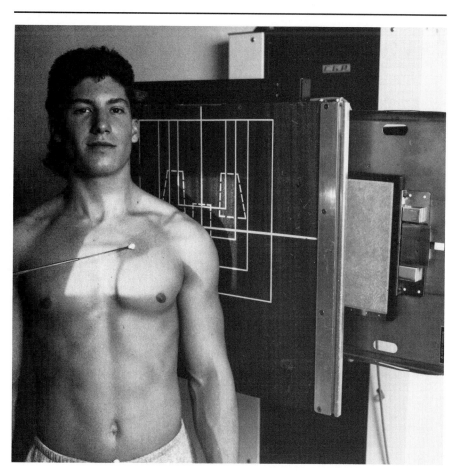

FIGURE 3-6　AP scapular plane position.

SHOULDER

LATERAL SCAPULAR PLANE POSITION

Pathology Demonstrated. Dislocation of the shoulder.

It is necessary to demonstrate the glenohumeral joint in a true lateral position to properly assess possible shoulder dislocation. However, many routine methods used to demonstrate the shoulder in the lateral position do not demonstrate the glenohumeral joint in a true lateral position. Neer and Rockwood[11] indicate a method of obtaining a true lateral position of the shoulder joint (Figure 3-7).

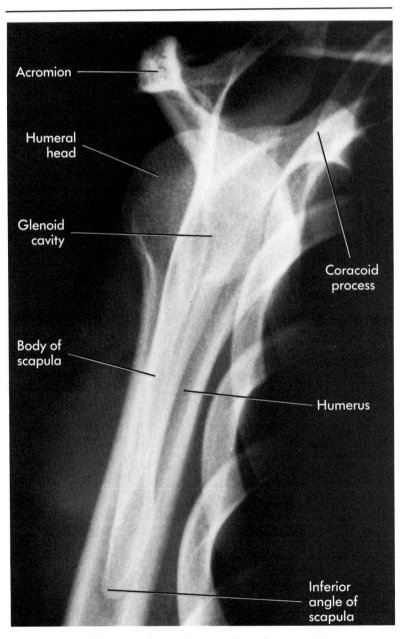

Acromion

Humeral head

Glenoid cavity

Coracoid process

Body of scapula

Humerus

Inferior angle of scapula

FIGURE 3-7   Lateral scapular plane position.

Patient Position. The patient should be standing or sitting facing the upright film-holding device which holds the cassette.

Part Position. To demonstrate the left side the patient should be positioned in a 45-degree LAO. To demonstrate the right side the patient should be positioned in a 45-degree RAO (Figure 3-8). The affected arm should be adducted to the side of the patient.

Central Ray. The central ray should be perpendicular to the film and directed to enter at the midpoint of the vertebral border of the scapula.

Radiograph Evaluation. The scapula should be demonstrated in a true lateral position.

The coracoid process, acromion, and the body of the scapula should be superimposed over the humerus and should appear as a Y.

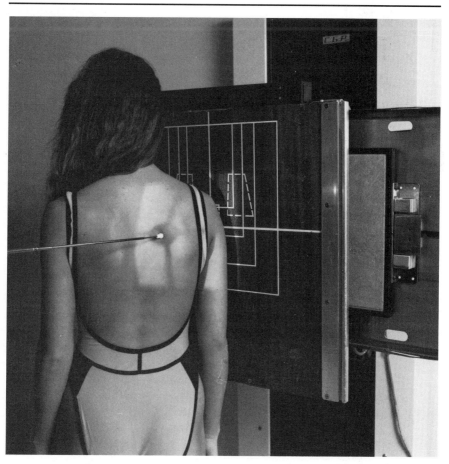

FIGURE 3-8   Lateral scapular plane position.

AP OBLIQUE POSITION

Pathology Demonstrated. Osteophyte formation on the inferior surfaces of the coracoid process and clavicle.

Bigliani and Morrison[1] indicate that osteophyte formation can occur as a result of osteoarthritis and may appear in the shoulder. Routine shoulder radiography does not adequately demonstrate the inferior surfaces of the clavicle or coracoid process, or of the osteophytes present there. An AP oblique position of the shoulder is useful for this purpose (Figure 3-9).

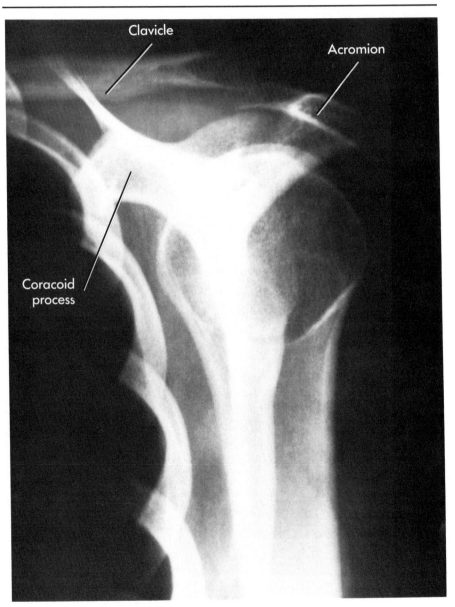

FIGURE 3-9   AP oblique position.

Patient Position. The patient should be standing or sitting with the back against the upright film-holding device which holds the cassette.

Part Position. To demonstrate the right side the patient should be positioned in a 45-degree LPO. To demonstrate the left side the patient should be positioned in a 45-degree RPO (Figure 3-10). The affected arm should be adducted to the side of the body.

Central Ray. The central ray should be angled 10 degrees cephalad and directed to enter at the medial portion of the humeral head.

Radiograph Evaluation. The shoulder should appear somewhat magnified.

The inferior surfaces of the coracoid process and clavicle should be well visualized.

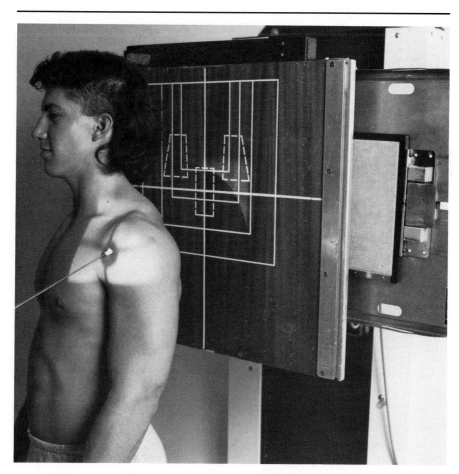

FIGURE 3-10   AP oblique position.

PA AXIAL POSITION: HERMODSSON'S METHOD

Pathology Demonstrated. Hill-Sachs defect.

The Hill-Sachs defect is a notch or depression of the posterolateral aspect of the humeral head created by the anterior margin of the glenoid rim after anterior dislocation of the shoulder has occurred. Neer and Rockwood[11] indicate that the Hill-Sachs defect is actually a compression fracture of this part of the humeral head and is generally larger in cases of recurrent anterior dislocation. Comparison views of both shoulders might be valuable in assessing Hill-Sachs defects.

There are several methods of identifying Hill-Sachs defects. Moseley[10] indicates that Hermodsson's method is useful for demonstrating this aspect of the humerus (Figure 3-11).

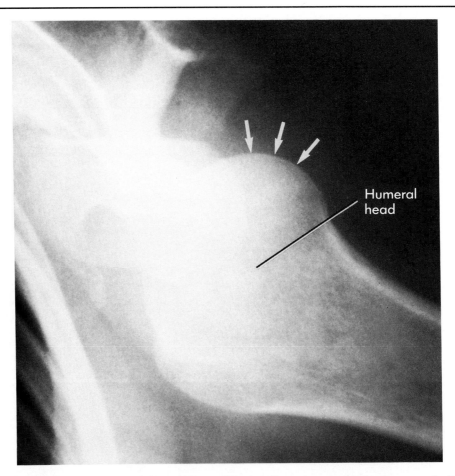

FIGURE 3-11   PA axial position: Hermodsson's method. Arrows indicate posterolateral aspect of humeral head.

Patient Position. The patient should be prone on the radiographic table with the cassette in the Bucky tray.

Part Position. The affected arm should be positioned to lie across the back. The hand should be positioned over the superior portion of the lumbar spine with the palmar surface facing up (Figure 3-12).

Central Ray. The central ray should be angled 30 degrees cephalad and directed to enter at the humeral head.

Radiograph Evaluation. The posterolateral aspect of the humeral head should be demonstrated in profile.

The humeral head should appear somewhat elongated.

The bony trabeculae of the posterolateral aspect of the humeral head should be well visualized.

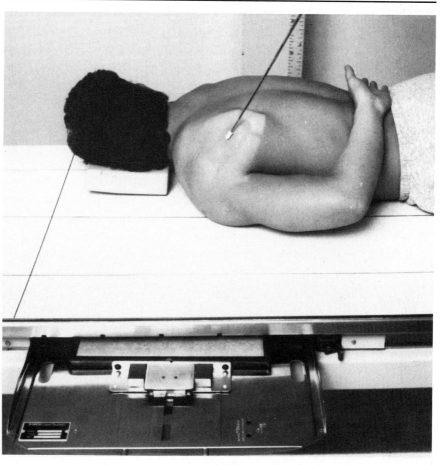

FIGURE 3-12   PA axial position: Hermodsson's method.

SHOULDER

PA AXIAL POSITION: DIDIEE METHOD

Pathology Demonstrated. Hill-Sachs defect.

Another method of demonstrating the Hill-Sachs defect is the Didiee method. Didiee[4] and Moseley[10] each indicate that this method is useful for demonstrating the posterolateral aspect of the humerus for this purpose (Figure 3-13).

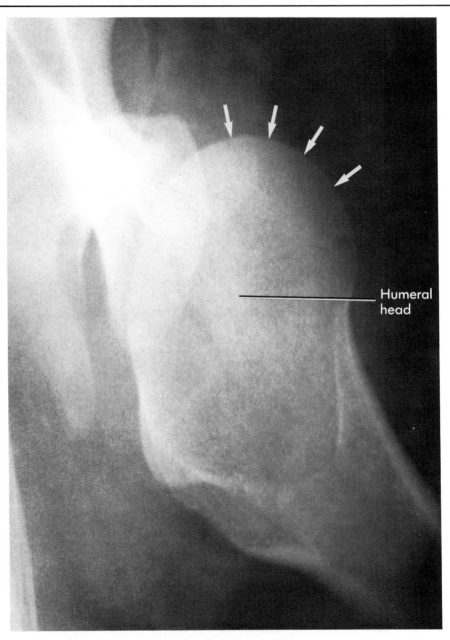

Humeral head

FIGURE 3-13   PA axial position: Didiee method. Arrows indicate posterolateral aspect of humeral head.

Patient Position. The patient should be prone on the radiographic table with the cassette in the Bucky tray.

Part Position. The affected arm should be positioned to lie across the back. The hand should be positioned over the superior portion of the lumbar spine with the palmar surface of the hand facing up (Figure 3-14).

Central Ray. The central ray should be angled 45 degrees cephalad and directed to enter at the humeral head.

Radiograph Evaluation. The posterolateral aspect of the humeral head should be demonstrated in profile.

The humeral head should appear somewhat elongated.

The bony trabeculae of the posterolateral aspect of the humeral head should be well visualized.

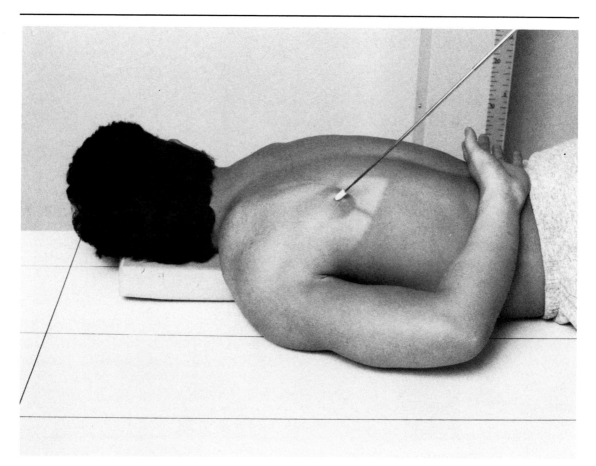

FIGURE 3-14   PA axial position: Didiee method.

SHOULDER

AP AXIAL POSITION: HERMODSSON'S INTERNAL ROTATION METHOD

Pathology Demonstrated. Hill-Sachs defect.

Hermodsson's internal rotation method will also demonstrate the Hill-Sachs defect. Hermodsson[6] indicates that this method of internal rotation of the humerus is useful for demonstrating the posterolateral aspect of the humerus for this purpose (Figure 3-15).

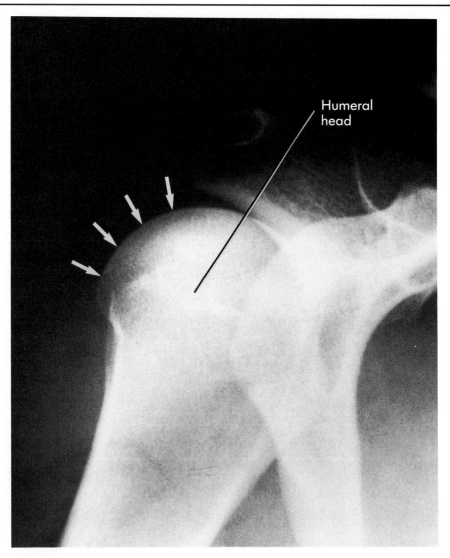

FIGURE 3-15 AP axial position: Hermodsson's internal rotation method. Arrows indicate posterolateral aspect of humeral head.

Patient Position. The patient should be supine on the radiographic table with the cassette in the Bucky tray.

Part Position. The affected arm should be positioned across the trunk with the dorsal surface of the hand facing up. Supporting devices, such as sponges, should be placed under the upper arm to position the humerus parallel with the radiographic tabletop (Figure 3-16).

Central Ray. The central ray should be angled 15 degrees caudad and directed to enter at the humeral head.

Radiograph Evaluation. The posterolateral aspect of the humerus should be demonstrated in profile.

The bony trabeculae of the posterolateral aspect of the humerus should be well visualized.

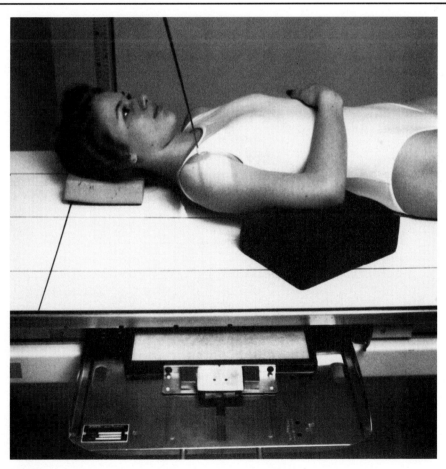

FIGURE 3-16 AP axial position: Hermodsson's internal rotation method.

AP 30-DEGREE AXIAL POSITION

Pathology Demonstrated. Hill-Sachs defect.

Matsen[9] indicates that an AP axial position of the shoulder is useful for demonstrating the posterolateral aspect of the humerus to identify a Hill-Sachs defect (Figure 3-17).

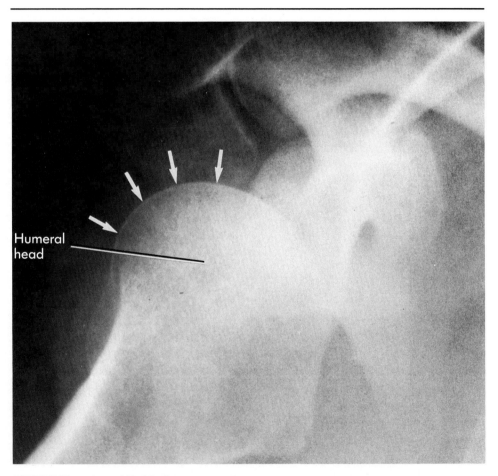

Humeral
head

FIGURE 3-17   AP 30-degree axial position. Arrows indicate posterolateral aspect of humeral head.

Patient Position. The patient should be supine on the radiographic table with the cassette in the Bucky tray.

Part Position. The affected arm should be slightly abducted and internally rotated (Figure 3-18).

Central Ray. The central ray should be angled 30 degrees caudad and directed to enter at the humeral head.

Radiograph Evaluation. The posterolateral aspect of the humeral head should be demonstrated in profile.

The humeral head should appear somewhat elongated.

The bony trabeculae of the posterolateral aspect of the humeral head should be well visualized.

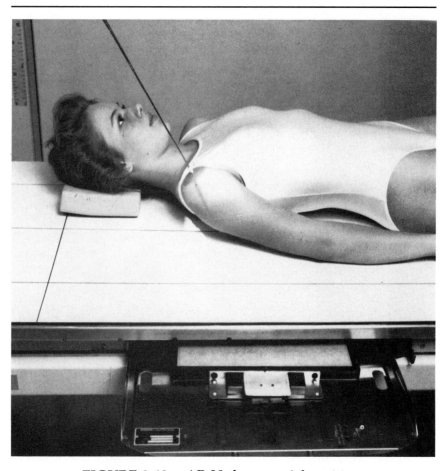

FIGURE 3-18   AP 30-degree axial position.

AP AXIAL POSITION: 10-DEGREE STRYKER METHOD

Pathology Demonstrated. Hill-Sachs defect.

Another method for demonstrating the Hill-Sachs defect exists. Hall, Isaac, and Booth[5] indicate that this method is useful for demonstrating the posterolateral aspect of the humeral head for this purpose (Figure 3-19).

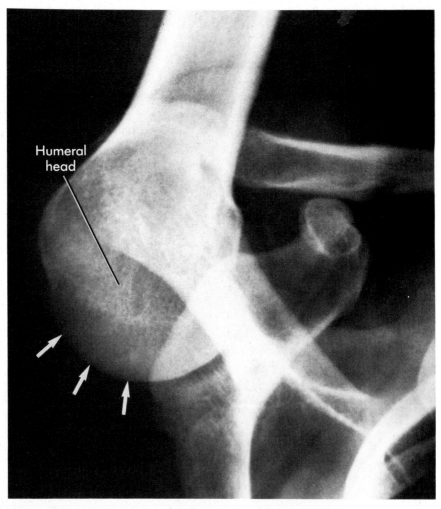

FIGURE 3-19 AP axial position: 10-degree Stryker method. Arrows indicate posterolateral aspect of humeral head.

Patient Position. The patient should be supine on the radiographic table with the cassette in the Bucky tray.

Part Position. The affected arm should be positioned so that the palmar surface of the hand rests on top of the head with the elbow pointing up (Figure 3-20).

Central Ray. The central ray should be angled 10 degrees cephalad and directed to enter at the humeral head.

Radiograph Evaluation. The posterolateral aspect of the humeral head should be demonstrated in profile.

   The bony trabeculae of the posterolateral aspect of the humeral head should be well visualized.

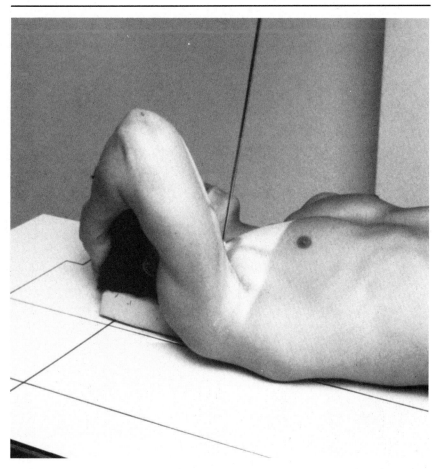

FIGURE 3-20   AP axial position: 10-degree Stryker method.

SHOULDER

AP AXIAL POSITION: WEST POINT METHOD–HILL-SACHS VARIATION

Pathology Demonstrated. Hill-Sachs defect.

A final method for demonstrating the Hill-Sachs defect is the West Point method–Hill-Sachs variation. This method is useful for demonstrating the posterolateral aspect of the humeral head for this purpose (Figure 3-21).

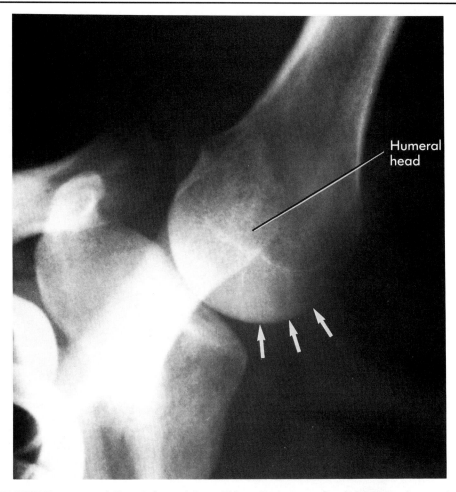

Humeral head

FIGURE 3-21 AP axial position: West Point method–Hill-Sachs variation. Arrows indicate posterolateral aspect of humeral head.

Patient Position. The patient should be standing or sitting with the back against the upright film-holding device which holds the cassette.

Part Position. The affected arm should be positioned so that the palmar surface of the hand is placed over the inferior portion of the cervical spine. The arm should be adducted to the side of the neck (Figure 3-22).

Central Ray. The central ray should be angled 10 degrees cephalad and directed to enter at the axilla.

Radiograph Evaluation. The posterolateral aspect of the humeral head should be demonstrated in profile.

The bony trabeculae of the posterolateral aspect of the humeral head should be well visualized.

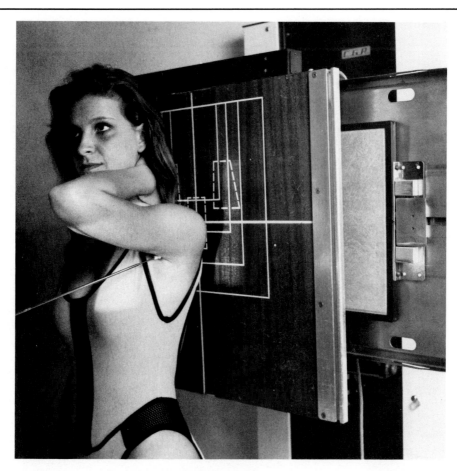

FIGURE 3-22   AP axial position: West Point method–Hill-Sachs variation.

SHOULDER

SUPRASPINATUS, INFRASPINATUS, AND TERES MINOR INSERTIONS: AP AXIAL POSITION

Pathology Demonstrated. Calcification of the supraspinatus, infraspinatus, and teres minor tendons.

The supraspinatus, infraspinatus, and teres minor muscles are inserted at the greater tubercle (tuberosity) of the humeral head. The greater tubercle must be radiographically demonstrated to assess calcific tendinitis at the site of insertion of these three muscles. Bigliani and Morrison[1] indicate that calcific tendinitis occurs most frequently in the shoulder in the supraspinatus tendon, second most frequently in the infraspinatus tendon, and somewhat less frequently in the teres minor tendon. Swallow and others[12] indicate a method that is useful for demonstrating the greater tubercle of the humeral head for this purpose (Figure 3-23).

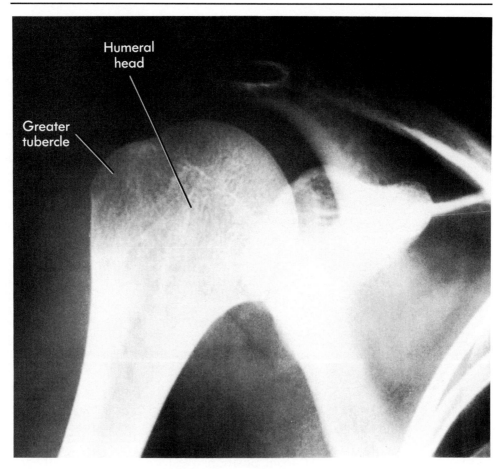

FIGURE 3-23 AP axial position.

Patient Position. The patient should be supine on the radiographic table with the cassette in the Bucky tray.

Part Position. The affected arm should be slightly abducted and supinated (Figure 3-24).

Central Ray. The central ray should be angled 25 degrees caudad and directed to enter at the humeral head.

Radiograph Evaluation. The greater tubercle of the humeral head should be demonstrated in profile.

The soft tissue surrounding the greater tubercle should be well visualized.

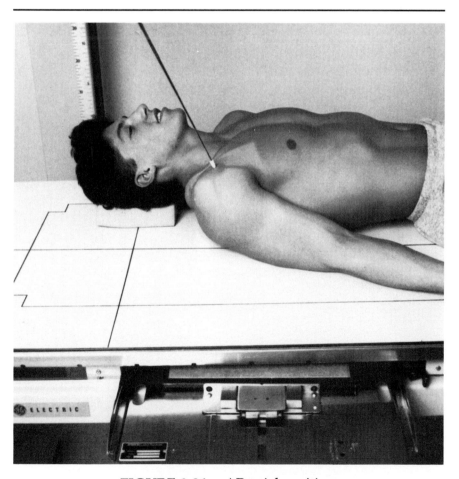

FIGURE 3-24 AP axial position.

SUBSCAPULARIS INSERTION: AP PROJECTION

Pathology Demonstrated. Calcification of the subscapularis tendon.

The subscapularis muscle is inserted at the lesser tubercle (tuberosity) of the humeral head. The lesser tubercle must be radiographically demonstrated to assess calcific tendinitis at the site of insertion of this muscle. Swallow and others[12] indicate a method that is useful for demonstrating the lesser tubercle of the humeral head for this purpose (Figure 3-25).

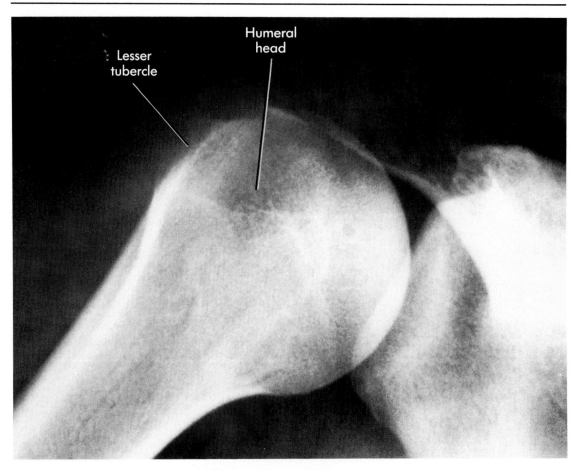

Lesser tubercle

Humeral head

FIGURE 3-25 AP projection.

Patient Position. The patient should be supine on the radiographic table with the cassette in the Bucky tray.

Part Position. The affected arm should be positioned so that the humerus is abducted and at a 45- to 90-degree angle to the body. The elbow should be flexed 90 degrees, and the dorsal surface of the hand should rest on the radiographic tabletop (Figure 3-26).

Central Ray. The central ray should be directed perpendicular to the film and directed to enter at the humeral head.

Radiograph Evaluation. The lesser tubercle of the humeral head should be demonstrated in profile.

The soft tissue surrounding the lesser tubercle should be well visualized.

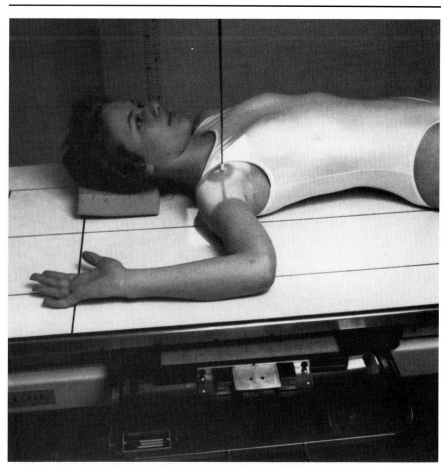

FIGURE 3-26 AP projection.

BICEPS INSERTION: AP PROJECTION

Pathology Demonstrated. Calcification of the biceps tendon.

Calcific tendinitis of the biceps tendon is often difficult to visualize because of the superimposition of other structures over the intertubercular (bicipital) groove. The method presented is used to demonstrate the intertubercular groove in profile for this purpose (Figure 3-27).

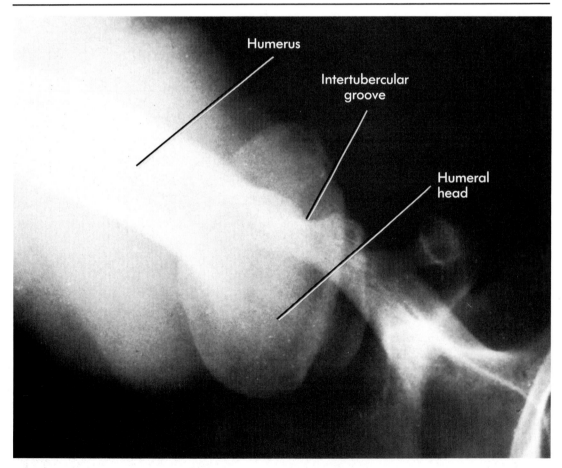

FIGURE 3-27   AP projection.

Patient Position. The patient should be supine on the radiographic table with the cassette in the Bucky tray.

Part Position. The affected arm should be positioned so that the palmar surface of the hand rests on top of the head with the elbow pointing up (Figure 3-28).

Central Ray. The central ray should be directed perpendicular to the film to enter at the humeral head.

Radiograph Evaluation. The intertubercular groove should be demonstrated in profile.

The soft tissue of the intertubercular groove should be well visualized.

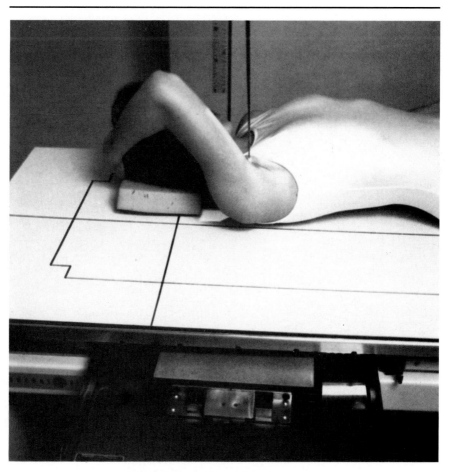

FIGURE 3-28   AP projection.

AP CORACOID POSITION

Pathology Demonstrated. Fracture of the coracoid process.

Routine methods of radiographing the shoulder demonstrate the coracoid process superimposed upon itself, which makes assessment of coracoid fracture difficult. Swallow and others[12] indicate a method for demonstrating the coracoid process free of superimposition for this purpose (Figure 3-29).

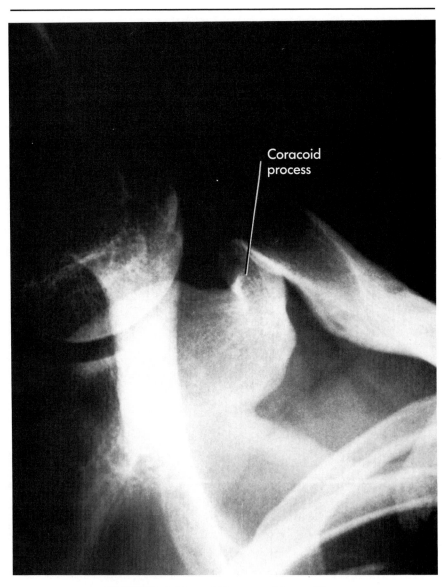

FIGURE 3-29 AP coracoid position.

Patient Position. The patient should be supine on the radiographic table with the cassette in the Bucky tray.

Part Position. To demonstrate the left side the patient should be positioned in a 10-degree RPO. To demonstrate the right side the patient should be positioned in a 10-degree LPO (Figure 3-30). The affected arm should be abducted and positioned so that the hand lies superior to the patient's head.

Central Ray. The central ray should be directed perpendicular to the film to enter 1 inch (3 cm) medial to the humeral head.

Radiograph Evaluation. The coracoid process should be demonstrated in profile.
    The coracoid process should not be superimposed upon itself.
    The bony trabeculae of the coracoid process should be well visualized.

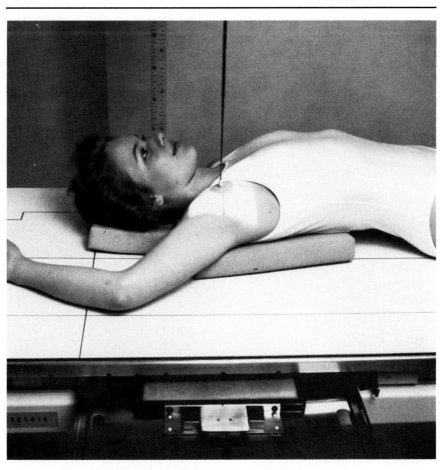

FIGURE 3-30   AP coracoid position.

AP AXIAL POSITION: 45-DEGREE STRYKER METHOD

Pathology Demonstrated. Fracture of the rim of the glenoid cavity (fossa).

Very little of the rim of the glenoid cavity can be seen on routine radiographs of the shoulder, which makes fracture assessment of this area of the shoulder difficult. McInnes[8] indicates a method that demonstrates approximately two thirds of the glenoid rim for this purpose (Figure 3-31).

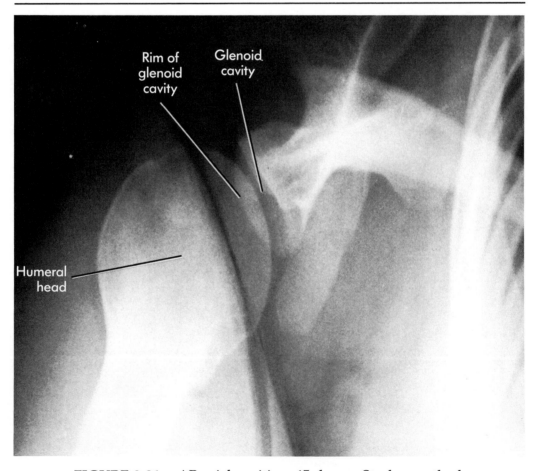

FIGURE 3-31   AP axial position: 45-degree Stryker method.

Patient Position. The patient should be supine on the radiographic table with the cassette in the Bucky tray.

Part Position. The affected arm should be slightly abducted and supinated (Figure 3-32).

Central Ray. The central ray should be angled 45 degrees caudad and directed to enter at the glenoid cavity.

Radiograph Evaluation. Approximately two thirds of the glenoid cavity should be demonstrated.

The glenoid cavity should be somewhat elongated and partially superimposed by the humeral head.

The bony trabeculae of the glenoid cavity and humeral head should be well visualized.

SHOULDER

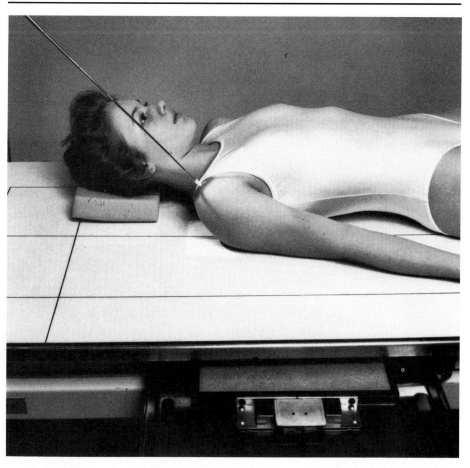

FIGURE 3-32   AP axial position: 45-degree Stryker method.

SUPINE OBLIQUE POSITION

Pathology Demonstrated. Fracture of the proximal humerus.

With patients who have experienced significant trauma, it is often difficult to radiographically demonstrate the proximal humerus in a lateral position for the purpose of demonstrating proximal humeral fractures. Transthoracic methods are useful in this area, but require that the patient be able to move the opposite upper limb to prevent significant superimposition. McInnes[8] indicates a method of demonstrating the proximal humerus in a nearly true lateral position that is achieved without having to move either upper limb and that is useful for this purpose (Figure 3-33).

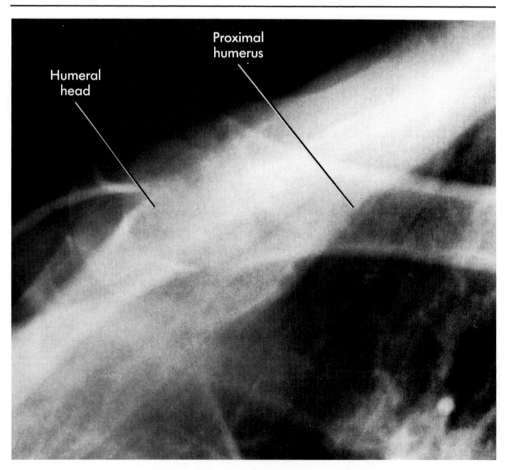

FIGURE 3-33   Supine oblique position.

Patient Position. The patient should be supine on the radiographic table or on a stretcher.

Part Position. To demonstrate the right side the patient should be positioned in a 10-degree LPO. To demonstrate the left side the patient should be positioned in a 10-degree RPO (Figure 3-34). The affected arm should be adducted to the side of the body. The film should be positioned vertically and in contact with the proximal upper limb.

Central Ray. The horizontal central ray should be directed perpendicular to the film to enter at the humeral head.

Radiograph Evaluation. The proximal portion of the humeral head should be demonstrated in a nearly true lateral position.

The affected proximal humerus should not be superimposed by the unaffected proximal humerus.

The proximal humerus should be adequately penetrated and the bony trabeculae somewhat visualized.

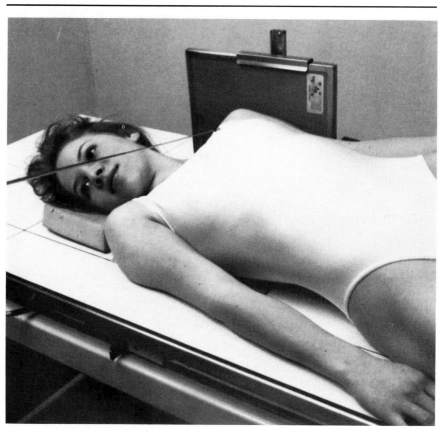

FIGURE 3-34   Supine oblique position.

❖ Acromioclavicular Joints

PA AXIAL OBLIQUE POSITION: ALEXANDER METHOD

Pathology Demonstrated. Acromioclavicular (AC) joint dislocation.

Routine methods used to demonstrate AC joint dislocation usually involve only AP projections in which exposures are made with the patient both holding weights and not holding weights. Neer and Rockwood[11] indicate a useful method of producing a lateral position of the AC joint (Figure 3-35) as an alternative to having the patient hold weights. If dislocation has occurred, the acromion will be displaced anteriorly and inferiorly under the lateral end of the clavicle.

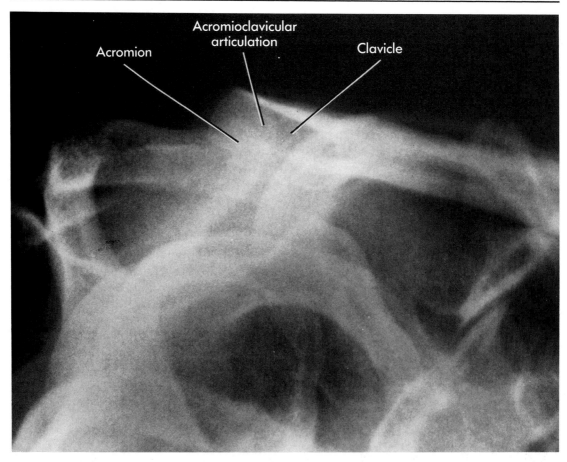

FIGURE 3-35   PA axial oblique position: Alexander method.

Patient Position. The patient should be standing or sitting and facing the upright film-holding device, which holds the cassette.

Part Position. Comparison studies of the unaffected and affected sides should be performed. To demonstrate the left side the patient should be positioned in a 45-degree LAO. To demonstrate the right side the patient should be positioned in a 45-degree RAO (Figure 3-36). Both shoulders should be rolled forward.

Central Ray. The central ray should be angled 10 degrees caudad and directed to enter at the AC joint.

Radiograph Evaluation. The AC joint should be well visualized.

The articular surface of the lateral end of the clavicle should be demonstrated end on.

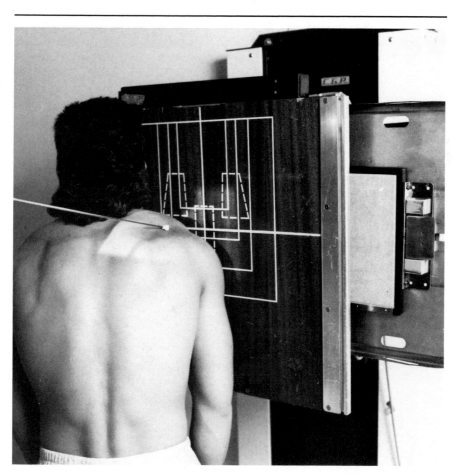

FIGURE 3-36   PA axial oblique position: Alexander method.

10-DEGREE AP AXIAL OBLIQUE POSITION

Pathology Demonstrated. Osteoarthritis of the acromioclavicular (AC) joint and osteophyte formation.

Bigliani and Morrison[1] indicate that when osteoarthritis or degenerative joint disease of the AC joint is present, there may also be osteophyte formation inferiorly. A special radiographic method is required to demonstrate the presence of both. A useful method for demonstrating both the AC joint in profile and the inferior surface of the AC joint and lateral end of the clavicle exists for this purpose (Figure 3-37).

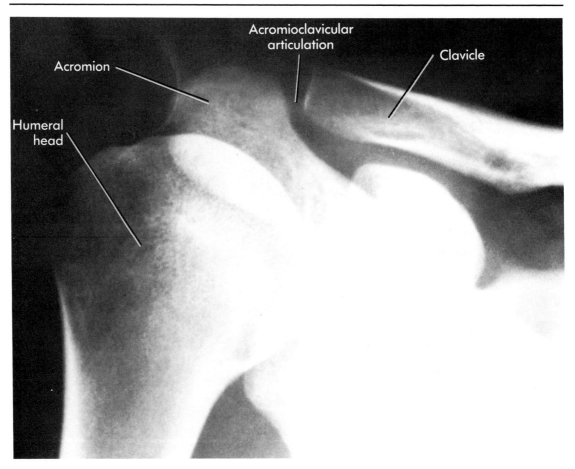

FIGURE 3-37   10-degree AP axial oblique position.

Patient Position. The patient should be standing or sitting with the back to the upright film-holding device which holds the cassette.

Part Position. To demonstrate the right side the patient should be positioned in a 10-degree RPO. To demonstrate the left side the patient should be positioned in a 10-degree LPO (Figure 3-38).

Central Ray. The central ray should be angled 10 degrees cephalad and directed to enter the AC joint.

Radiograph Evaluation. The AC joint should be demonstrated in profile.

The inferior surface of the AC joint and the lateral end of the clavicle should be well visualized.

The AC joint should be well visualized.

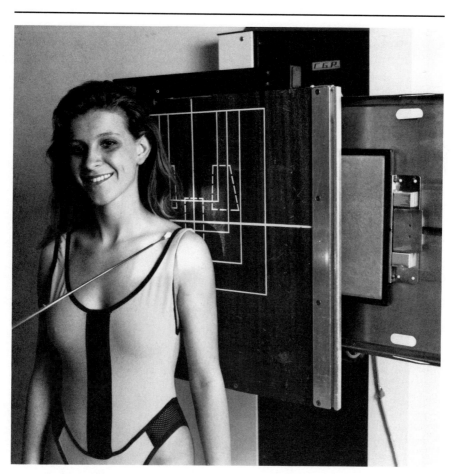

FIGURE 3-38 10-degree AP axial oblique position.

ACROMIOCLAVICULAR JOINTS

PA OBLIQUE POSITION

Pathology Demonstrated. Subacromial impingement syndrome.

Subacromial impingement syndrome is described by Bigliani and Morrison[1] as impingement of the rotator cuff, biceps tendon, and the subacromial bursa between the humeral head and the acromion when the affected arm is elevated. Impingement may be indicated by excrescence of the greater tubercle (tuberosity), osteophyte formation on the anterior surface of the acromion process and the inferior surface of the lateral end of the clavicle, and arthritis of the acromioclavicular (AC) joint. A useful method exists for demonstrating each of these structures (Figure 3-39).

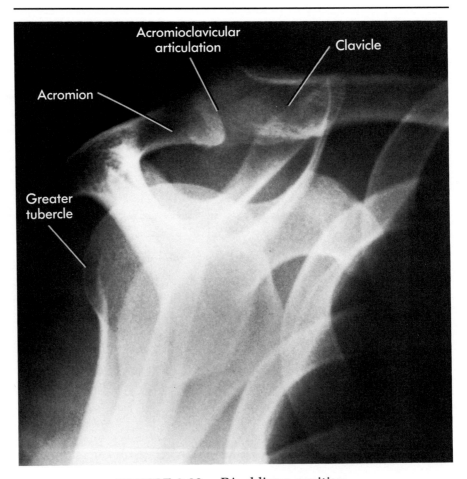

FIGURE 3-39   PA oblique position.

Patient Position. The patient should be standing or sitting upright and facing the upright film-holding device which holds the cassette.

Part Position. The affected arm should be positioned in neutral rotation. To demonstrate the left side the patient should be positioned in a 45-degree LAO. To demonstrate the right side the patient should be positioned in a 45-degree RAO (Figure 3-40).

Central Ray. The horizontal central ray should be directed to enter the space between the humeral head and acromion.

Radiograph Evaluation. The space between the humeral head and acromion should be demonstrated.

The greater tubercle of the humeral head should be demonstrated in profile.

The AC joint should be demonstrated.

The anterior surface of the acromion and the inferior surface of the lateral end of the clavicle should be demonstrated.

The bony trabeculae of the greater tubercle, the acromion, and the clavicle should be well visualized.

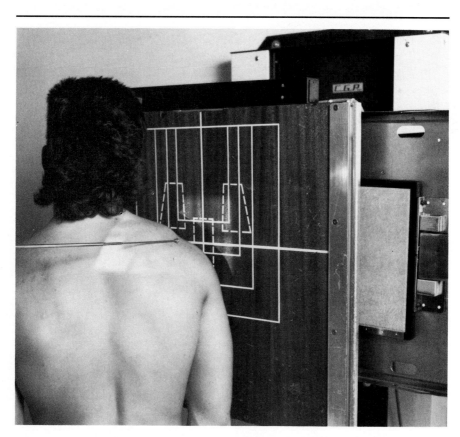

FIGURE 3-40   PA oblique position.

PA AXIAL OBLIQUE POSITION

Pathology Demonstrated. Osteophyte formation on the inferior surfaces of the lateral end of the clavicle and the acromion.

This method is useful for demonstrating the inferior surfaces of the lateral end of the clavicle and the acromion (Figure 3-41).

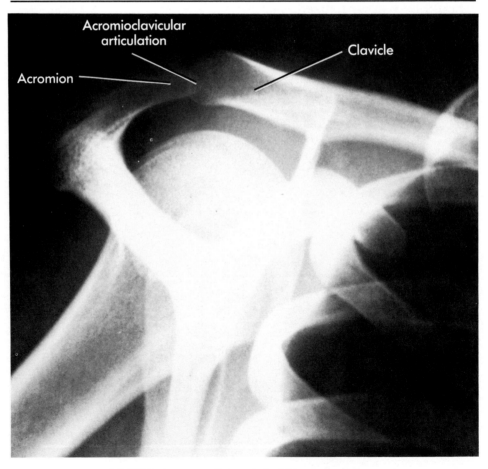

FIGURE 3-41   PA axial oblique position.

Patient Position. The patient should be standing or sitting upright and facing the upright film-holding device which holds the cassette.

Part Position. The affected hand should be positioned on the hip, and the unaffected hand should be positioned to hold the top of the upright film-holding device. To demonstrate the left side the patient should be positioned in a 45-degree LAO. To demonstrate the right side the patient should be positioned in a 45-degree RAO (Figure 3-42).

Central Ray. The central ray should be angled 15 degrees caudad and directed to enter at the acromioclavicular joint.

Radiograph Evaluation. The inferior surfaces of the acromion and lateral end of the clavicle should be demonstrated.

The acromion and lateral end of the clavicle should form an arch superior to the humeral head.

The bony trabeculae of the acromion and clavicle should be well visualized.

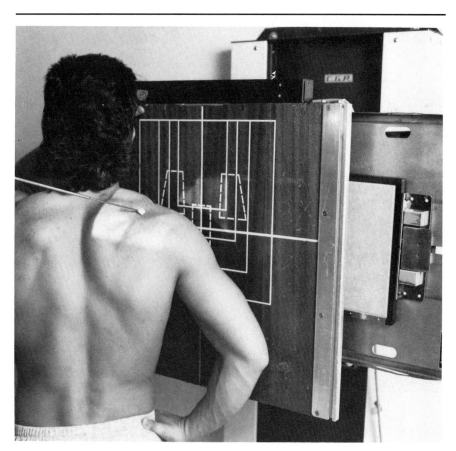

FIGURE 3-42 PA axial oblique position.

ACROMIOCLAVICULAR JOINTS

CHAPTER 3 • REFERENCES

1. Bigliani LU, Morrison DS: *Miscellaneous degenerative disorders of the shoulder.* In Dee RD, Mango E, Hurst LC, editors: *Principles of orthopaedic practice,* vol 1, New York, 1989, McGraw-Hill.

2. Bloom MH, Obata WG: Diagnosis of posterior dislocation of the shoulder with use of Velpeau axillary and angle-up roentgenographic views, *J Bone Joint Surg* 49A:943, 1967.

3. Ciullo JV, Koniuch MP, Teitge RA: C.A.M. axillary x-ray exhibit to the academy meeting of the American Academy of Orthopaedic Surgeons, *Orthop Trans* 6:451, 1982.

4. Didiee J: Radiodiagnostic dans la luxation recidivante de l'epaule, *J Radiol Electrol* 14:191, 1929.

5. Hall RH, Isaac F, Booth CR: Dislocation of the shoulder with special reference to accompanying small fractures, *J Bone Joint Surg* 41A:489, 1959.

6. Hermodsson I: Rontgenologische studein uber die traumatischen und habituellen schultergelenk-verrenkungen nach vorn und nach unten, *Acta Radiol* 20(suppl):1, 1934.

7. Hill HA, Sachs MD: The grooved defect of the humeral head: a frequently unrecognized complication of dislocations of the shoulder joint, *Radiology* 35:690, 1940.

8. McInnes J: *Clark's positioning in radiography,* ed 9, vol 1, Chicago, 1973, Mosby–Year Book.

9. Matsen FA III: *The shoulder, arm and elbow.* In Evarts CM, editor: *Surgery of the musculoskeletal system,* vol 3, New York, 1983, Churchill Livingstone.

10. Moseley HF: *Recurrent dislocation of the shoulder,* Montreal, 1961, McGill University Press.

11. Neer CS II, Rockwood CA Jr: *Fractures and dislocations of the shoulder.* In Rockwood CA Jr., Green DP, editors: *Fractures in adults,* ed 2, Philadelphia, 1984, JB Lippincott.

12. Swallow RA, Naylor E, Whitley AS, and others: *Clark's positioning in radiography,* ed 11, Rockville, Md, 1986, Aspen.

CHAPTER
4
The Bony Thorax

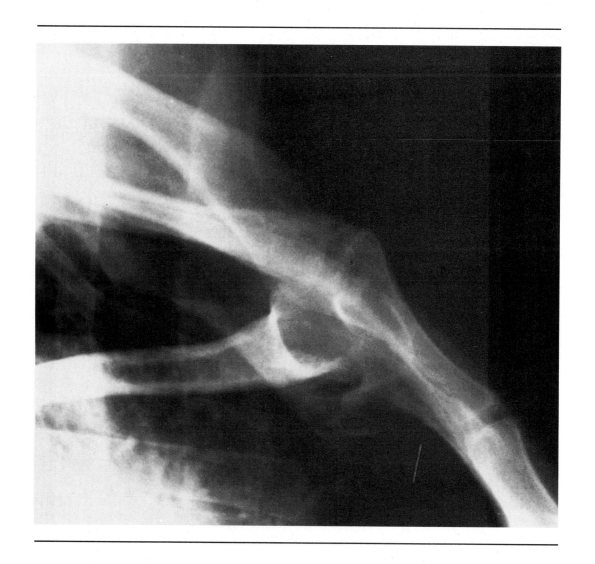

STERNOCLAVICULAR JOINTS

❖ Sternoclavicular Joints

AP AXIAL POSITION

Pathology Demonstrated. Dislocation of the sternoclavicular (SC) joints.

Dislocation of the SC joints is often difficult to assess with routine methods. Neer and Rockwood[5] indicate a method that is useful for demonstrating SC joints. With this method, if no dislocation has occurred, then the medial ends of both clavicles should lie in the same horizontal plane (Figure 4-1). If anterior dislocation has occurred, the medial end of the dislocated clavicle is demonstrated superior to this plane. If posterior dislocation has occurred, the medial end of the dislocated clavicle is demonstrated inferior to this plane.

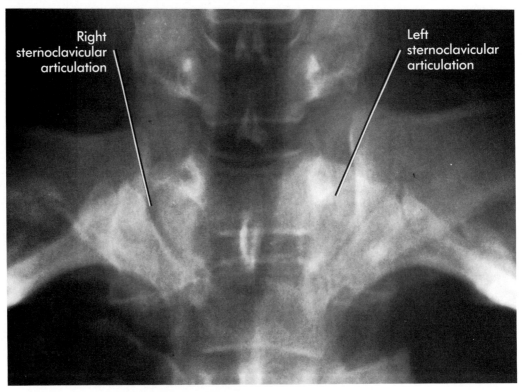

FIGURE 4-1   AP axial position.

Patient Position. The patient should be supine on the radiographic table with the cassette placed in the Bucky tray.

Part Position. The arms should be adducted to the patient's side (Figure 4-2).

Central Ray. The central ray should be angled 45 degrees cephalad and directed to enter the manubrium of the sternum.

Radiograph Evaluation. The SC joints should be demonstrated in profile.
    The medial ends of both clavicles should be somewhat elongated.
    The upper thorax should appear somewhat lordotic.
    The SC joints should be well visualized.

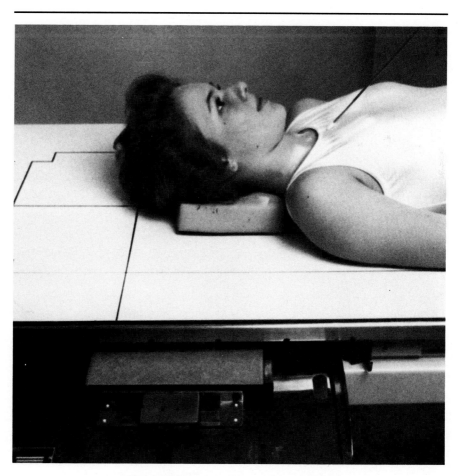

FIGURE 4-2   AP axial position.

STERNOCLAVICULAR JOINTS

PA AXIAL POSITION

Pathology Demonstrated. Dislocation of the sternoclavicular (SC) joints.

Another method for better demonstrating dislocation of the SC joints exists. Hobbs[3] indicates his alternative method for demonstrating the SC joints produces a result very similar to the AP axial position, but with less radiographic distortion. With this method if no dislocation has occurred, then the medial ends of both clavicles should lie in the same horizontal plane (Figure 4-3). If anterior dislocation has occurred, the medial end of the dislocated clavicle is demonstrated superior to this plane. If posterior dislocation has occurred, the medial end of the dislocated clavicle is demonstrated inferior to this plane.

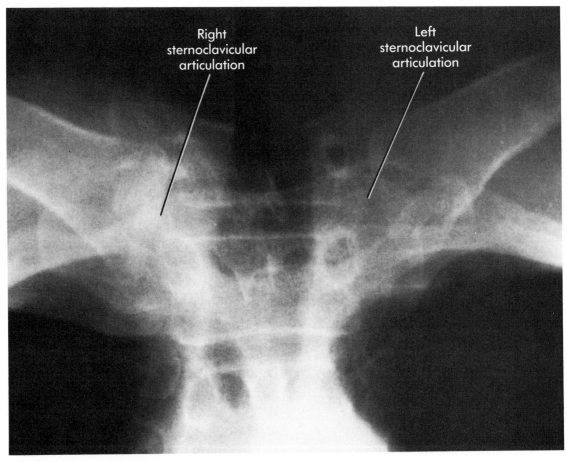

FIGURE 4-3   PA axial position.

Patient Position. The patient should be seated beside or at the end of the radiographic table.

Part Position. The cassette should be placed on the radiographic tabletop. The patient should be positioned so that the coronal plane of the thorax forms a 35- to 45-degree angle to the plane of the cassette. The SC joints should be positioned over the cassette, and the patient's hands wrapped around the back of the head. The patient's neck should be parallel to the cassette, and the arms should be adducted to the side of the head (Figure 4-4).

Central Ray. The central ray should be directed perpendicular to the film and directed to pass through the jugular (manubrial) notch.

Radiograph Evaluation. The SC joints should be demonstrated in profile.
    The medial ends of both clavicles should be somewhat elongated.
    The upper thorax should appear somewhat lordotic.
    The SC joints should be well visualized.

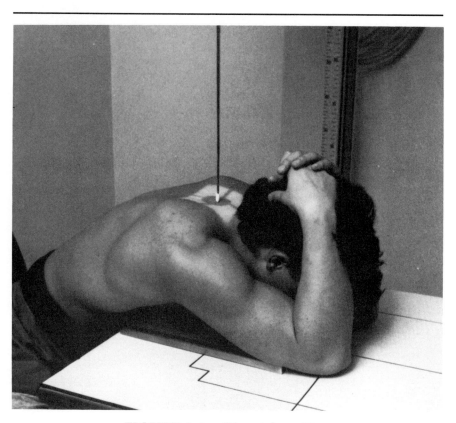

FIGURE 4-4   PA axial position.

STERNOCLAVICULAR JOINTS

STERNOCLAVICULAR JOINTS

LATERAL BENDING POSITION

Pathology Demonstrated. Dislocation of the sternoclavicular (SC) joints.

Anterior or posterior dislocation of the SC joints can also be demonstrated in a lateral position. Kimberlin[4] indicates a method that is useful for demonstrating the SC joints in a lateral position without superimposition of the medial ends of the clavicles (Figure 4-5). If anterior dislocation has occurred, the medial end of the dislocated clavicle is demonstrated more anterior than the normal clavicle. If posterior dislocation has occurred, the medial end of the dislocated clavicle is demonstrated more posterior than the normal clavicle.

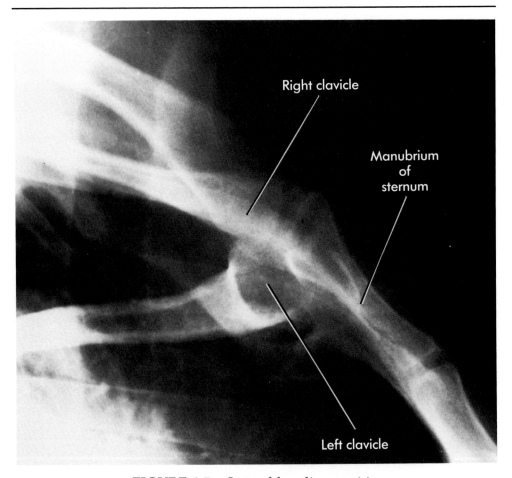

FIGURE 4-5   Lateral bending position.

Patient Position. The patient should be standing or sitting with either side against the upright film-holding device which holds the cassette.

Part Position. The patient should be instructed to move one step away from the upright film-holding device and should be positioned to bend at the waist toward the upright film-holding device. The affected arm should be adducted to the side of the body and the unaffected arm extended above the head and holding the top of the upright film-holding device (Figure 4-6).

Central Ray. The horizontal central ray should be directed perpendicular to the film to enter at the jugular (manubrial) notch.

Radiograph Evaluation. The medial ends of both clavicles should be demonstrated.

The manubrium of the sternum should be demonstrated in a lateral position. The medial ends of the clavicles should be well visualized.

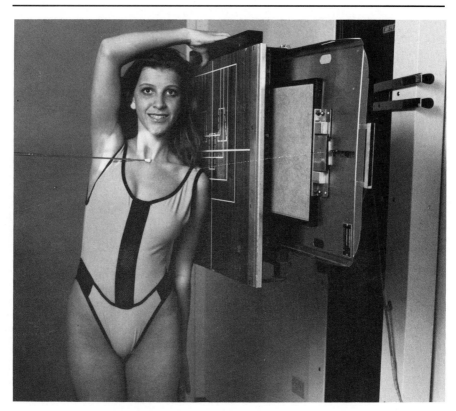

FIGURE 4-6   Lateral bending position.

STERNOCLAVICULAR JOINTS

PA AXIAL OBLIQUE POSITION: BARRONG METHOD

Pathology Demonstrated. Neoplasm or infection of the medial end of the clavicle and involving the sternoclavicular (SC) joint.

Almost all methods of radiographing the SC joints demonstrate the joints superimposed over several bony structures, such as ribs and the vertebral column. These methods are adequate to demonstrate dislocation of the SC joints but are poor for demonstrating any neoplastic process of the medial ends of the clavicles and SC joints. Barrong[1] indicates a method that is useful for this purpose and demonstrates the SC joints in profile and free of superimposition of the vertebral column (Figure 4-7).

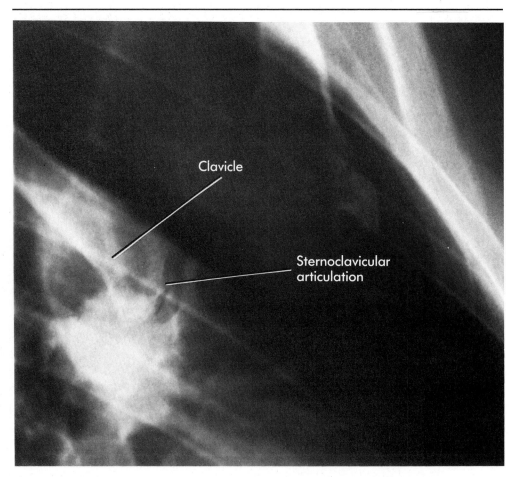

FIGURE 4-7　PA axial oblique position: Barrong method.

Patient Position. The patient should be prone on the radiographic table with the cassette placed in the Bucky tray.

Part Position. To demonstrate the right side the patient should be positioned in a 45-degree RAO. To demonstrate the left side the patient should be positioned in a 45-degree LAO (Figure 4-8).

Central Ray. The central ray should be angled 20 degrees cephalad and directed to pass through the affected SC joint.

Radiograph Evaluation. The affected SC joint should be demonstrated in profile. The affected SC joint should not be superimposed over the vertebral column. The bony trabeculae of the medial end of the clavicle should be well visualized. The affected SC joint should be well visualized.

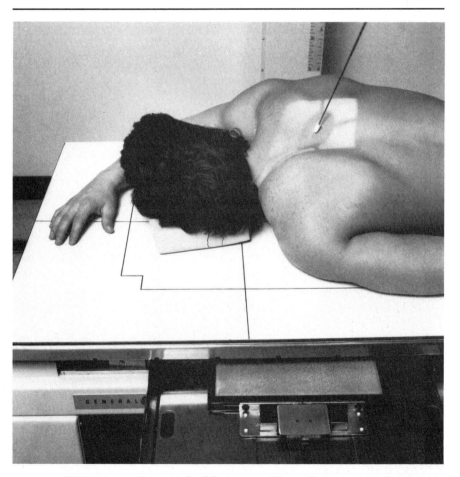

FIGURE 4-8 PA axial oblique position: Barrong method.

❖ Sternum

PA AXIAL POSITION

Pathology Demonstrated. Sternum fracture.

Radiography of the sternum can be difficult to perform on patients who are experiencing considerable pain. Pain in the area of the sternum can be intensified when routine methods are used to radiograph the sternum. Bull[2] indicates that this method is useful with ambulatory patients who are experiencing substantial pain (Figure 4-9).

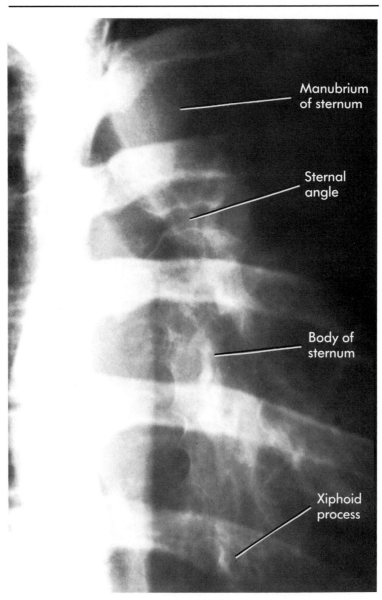

FIGURE 4-9   PA axial position.

Patient Position. The patient should be standing beside and facing the radiographic table with the cassette placed in the Bucky tray.

Part Position. The patient should bend at the waist with the thorax over the center of the table. The arms should be positioned superior to the shoulders with the palmar surfaces of the hands resting on the radiographic table; the patient should rest the head on both arms for comfort (Figure 4-10). The x-ray tube should be positioned to the right of the patient. A shallow breathing technique can be used to reduce the imaging of prominent pulmonary markings.

Central Ray. The central ray should be angled 25 degrees medially and directed to enter 2 inches (5 cm) lateral to the seventh thoracic vertebra. Large patients should be radiographed using a lesser angle; thin patients should be radiographed using a greater angle.

Radiograph Evaluation. The sternum should be demonstrated within the cardiac shadow.

Pulmonary markings should be blurred on the radiograph.

The sternum should be sufficiently well contrasted against surrounding structures.

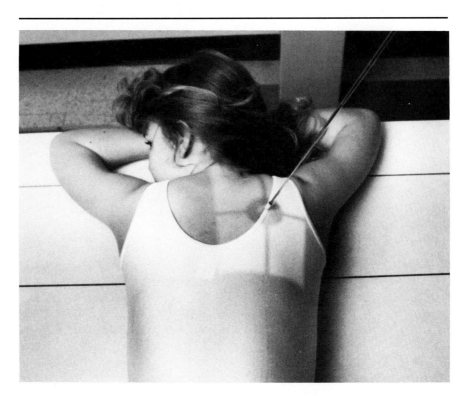

FIGURE 4-10 PA axial position.

STERNUM

COMPOSITE RAO POSITION

Pathology Demonstrated. Sternum fracture.

It is often difficult to produce a satisfactory radiograph of the sternum with the routine RAO position. Piotrowski[6] indicates a method that makes the routine RAO more useful for demonstrating the sternum by blurring the overlying ribs (Figure 4-11).

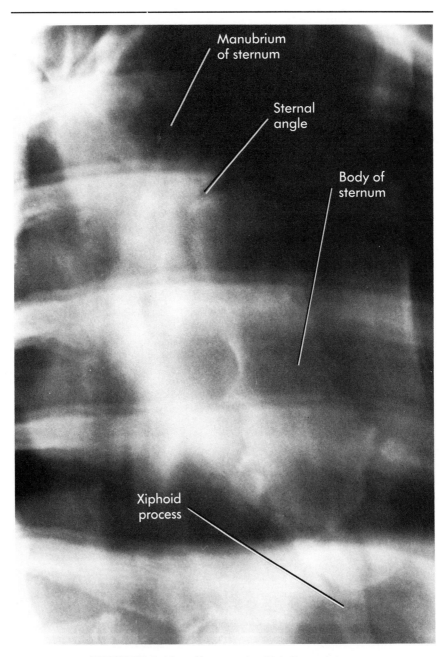

Manubrium of sternum

Sternal angle

Body of sternum

Xiphoid process

FIGURE 4-11 Composite RAO position.

Patient Position. The patient should be prone on the radiographic table with the cassette placed in the Bucky tray.

Part Position. The patient should be positioned in a 15- to 20-degree RAO position. Two exposures should be made on the same film, each using half the mAs normally used for an RAO sternum radiograph.

Central Ray. The central ray should be directed perpendicular to the film and directed to pass through the midsternum. For the first exposure the central ray should be angled 5 degrees cephalad without adjusting the position of the film or the patient (Figure 4-12). For the second exposure the central ray should be angled 5 degrees caudad without adjusting the position of the film or the patient (Figure 4-13). A shallow breathing technique can be used to prevent the imaging of prominent pulmonary markings.

Radiograph Evaluation. The sternum should be demonstrated within the cardiac shadow.

Ribs and pulmonary markings should be blurred on the radiograph.

The sternum should be sufficiently well contrasted against surrounding structures.

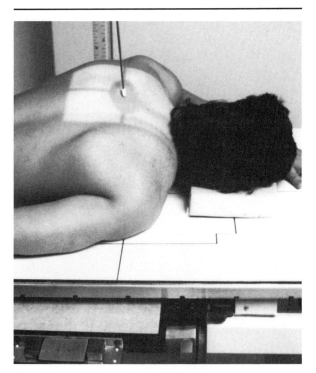

FIGURE 4-12 Composite RAO position with central ray angled 5 degrees cephalad.

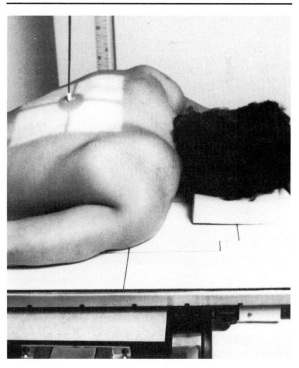

FIGURE 4-13 Composite RAO position with central ray angled 5 degrees caudad.

STERNUM

CHAPTER 4 • REFERENCES

1. Barrong WR: Radiography of the sternoclavicular articulation, *The x-ray technician, J Am Soc X-Ray Technicians* 25:368, Sept 1953.
2. Bull E: Technique for a true posteroanterior projection of the sternum and the sternoclavicular articulations, *The x-ray technician, J Am Soc X-Ray Technicians* 53:259, 1953.
3. Hobbs DW: Sternoclavicular joint: a new axial radiographic view, *Radiology* 90:801, 1968.
4. Kimberlin GE: Radiography of injuries to the region of the shoulder girdle: revisited, *Radiol Technol* 46:69, 1974.
5. Neer CS II, Rockwood CA Jr: *Fractures and dislocations of the shoulder.* In Rockwood CA Jr, Green DP, editors: *Fractures in adults,* ed 2, Philadelphia, 1984, JB Lippincott.
6. Piotrowski D: Helpful hints in radiographing the sternum, *The x-ray technician, J Am Soc X-Ray Technicians* 15:230, May 1944.

5

The Lower Limb (Foot and Ankle)

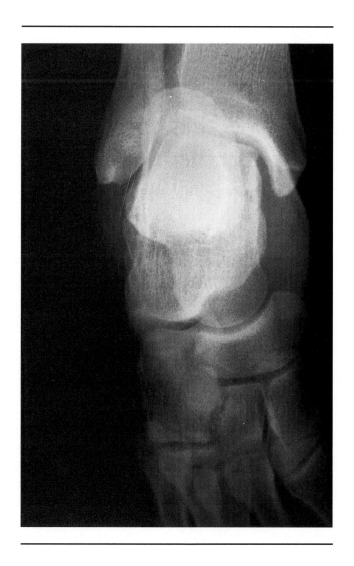

❖ Foot

AP AXIAL POSITION

Pathology Demonstrated. Fractures of the talus (astragalus) involving the articulation with the navicular (scaphoid) and fractures of the calcaneus (os calcis) involving the articulation with the cuboid.

Often, routine radiographic methods of the foot do not adequately demonstrate the talar neck and its articulation with the navicular or the anterior portion of the calcaneus and its articulation with the cuboid. There is a useful method (Figure 5-1) for demonstrating these areas of the foot.

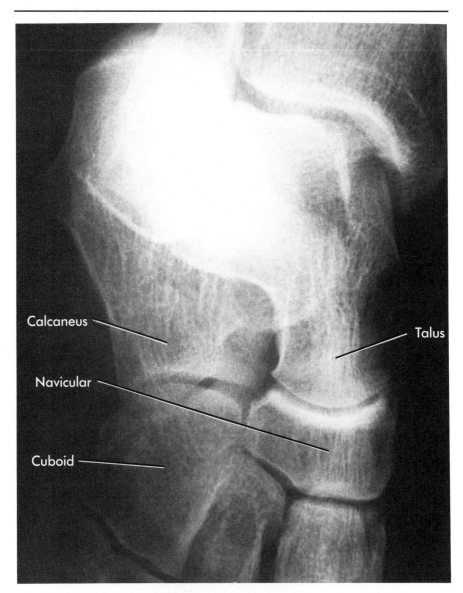

FIGURE 5-1   AP axial position.

Patient Position. The patient should be supine on the radiographic table. The affected knee should be flexed approximately 90 degrees to allow the plantar surface of the foot to lie flat on the cassette, which is placed on the radiographic tabletop.

Part Position. The affected leg should be positioned in maximum internal rotation with the foot remaining flat on the cassette (Figure 5-2).

Central Ray. The central ray should be angled 15 degrees posterior and directed to enter 1 inch (3 cm) anterior to the distal end of the fibula.

Radiographic Evaluation. The neck of the talus and its articulation with the navicular should be demonstrated.

The anterior portion of the calcaneus and its articulation with the cuboid should be demonstrated.

The talus and calcaneus should appear somewhat elongated.

The bony trabeculae of the talus and calcaneus should be well visualized.

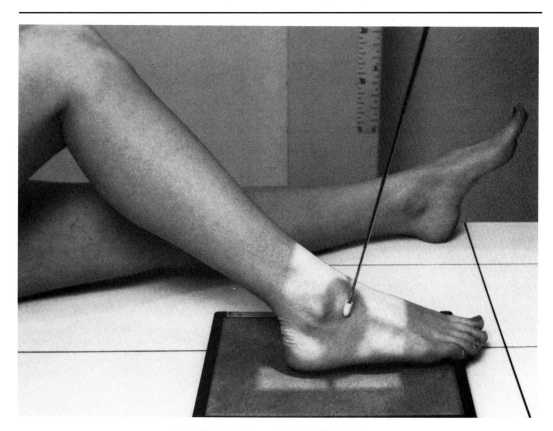

FIGURE 5-2   AP axial position.

BILATERAL LATERAL POSITIONS

Pathology Demonstrated. Presence and fracture of os trigonum near the talus (astragalus) or calcaneus (os calcis).

According to Heckman[3] os trigonum is the most frequently occurring of several accessory ossicles found in the foot and is of potential clinical importance in patients who are suspected of having either a talar or calcaneal fracture. That is, it is important to distinguish between the presence of os trigonum and the fracture of either the medial or lateral tubercles of the talus or the calcaneus, or the fracture of the os trigonum itself, if present. McInnes[4] indicates that the lateral position of the talus and calcaneus is useful for demonstrating os trigonum and that bilateral lateral positions (Figures 5-3 and 5-4) are useful for comparison of the affected side with the unaffected.

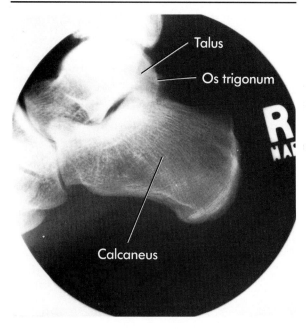

FIGURE 5-3   Lateral position.

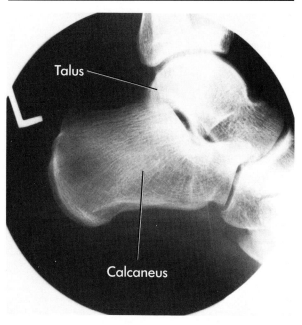

FIGURE 5-4   Lateral position.

Patient Position. Two lateral positions, one of each talus and calcaneus, should be obtained. To obtain the lateral position the patient should be placed in a lateral recumbent position with the limb of interest fully extended.

Part Position. The foot should be slightly dorsiflexed with the lateral surface of the foot in contact with the cassette, which is placed on the radiographic tabletop (Figure 5-5). The talus and calcaneus of the other limb should then be radiographed in the same manner (Figure 5-6).

Central Ray. The central ray should be directed perpendicular to the film to enter at the middle portion of the calcaneus.

Radiograph Evaluation. The talus and calcaneus of each foot should be demonstrated in the lateral position.

    The x-ray field should be tightly collimated to the anatomic part of interest.

    The bony trabeculae of the talus and calcaneus should be well visualized.

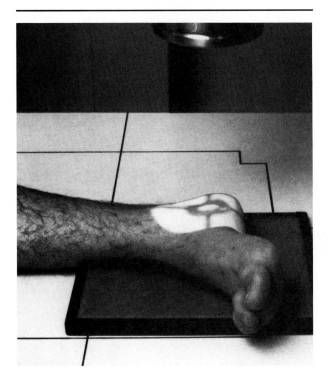

FIGURE 5-5   Lateral position.

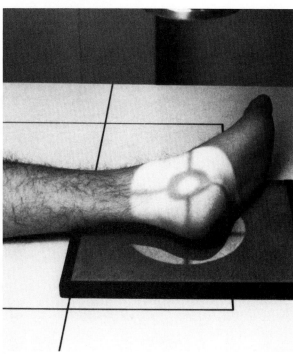

FIGURE 5-6   Lateral position.

FOOT

AP STRESS PROJECTION

Pathology Demonstrated. Persistent or recurrent joint incongruity or osseous instability.

Nonstress radiographs of the foot may not show persistent or recurring joint or bone problems following closed reduction of fractures or dislocations. Wilson[5] indicates that the AP projection of the foot with stress provided by gravity (Figure 5-7) is valuable for assessing the presence of recurrent joint incongruity or osseous instability.

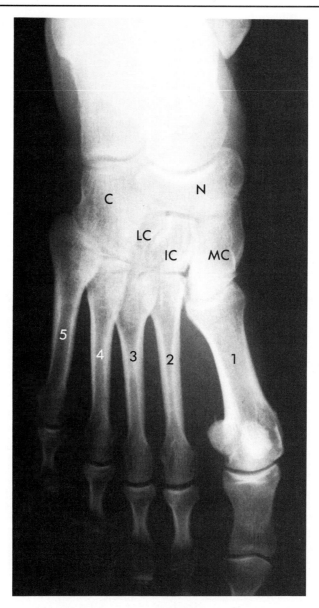

FIGURE 5-7 AP stress projection. The metatarsals are numbered 1 through 5. *MC*, medial cuneiform; *IC*, intermediate cuneiform; *LC*, lateral cuneiform; *C*, cuboid; *N*, navicular.

Patient Position. The patient should be seated on the radiographic table with the affected leg dangling over the side of the table.

Part Position. The affected foot should not be positioned but instead should be allowed to dangle freely. The radiographic cassette should be positioned under the plantar surface of the foot and parallel to it but not in contact with it (Figure 5-8). The cassette should be built-up off the floor to place it very close to the foot; this can be accomplished with a variety of available materials, including positioning sponges.

Central Ray. The central ray should be angled 10 degrees posteriorly and directed to enter at the base of the third metatarsal.

Radiograph Evaluation. The foot should be demonstrated without rotation.
The joints and bony trabeculae should be adequately visualized.

FOOT

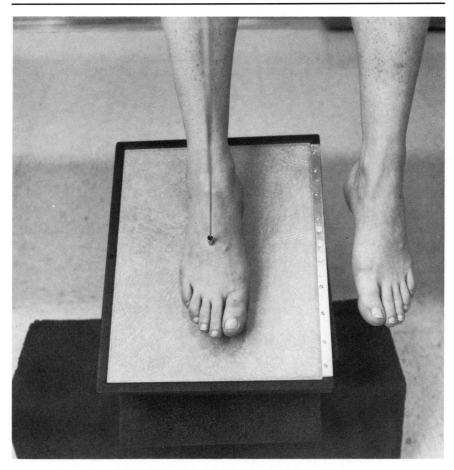

FIGURE 5-8   AP stress projection.

FOOT

LATERAL STRESS POSITION

Pathology Demonstrated. Persistent or recurrent joint incongruity or osseous instability.

Nonstress radiographs of the foot may not show persistent or recurring joint or bone problems following closed reduction of fractures or dislocations. Wilson[5] indicates that the lateral position of the foot with stress provided by gravity (Figure 5-9) is valuable for assessing the presence of recurrent joint incongruity or osseous instability.

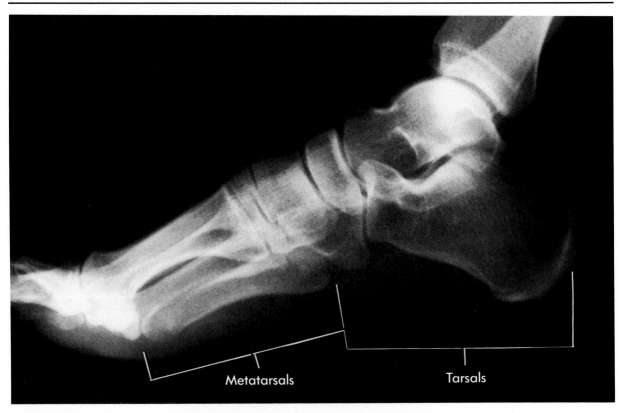

Metatarsals   Tarsals

FIGURE 5-9   Lateral stress position.

Patient Position. The patient should be seated on the radiographic table with the affected leg dangling over the side of the table.

Part Position. The affected foot should not be positioned but instead should be allowed to dangle freely. The radiographic cassette should be positioned beside the medial surface of the foot and parallel to it (Figure 5-10). The cassette should be built-up from the floor to place the cassette very close to the foot; this can be accomplished with a variety of available materials, including positioning sponges.

Central Ray. The central ray should be directed perpendicular to the cassette to enter at the base of the third metatarsal.

Radiograph Evaluation. The foot should be demonstrated in a lateral position without rotation.

The joints and bony trabeculae should be adequately visualized.

FOOT

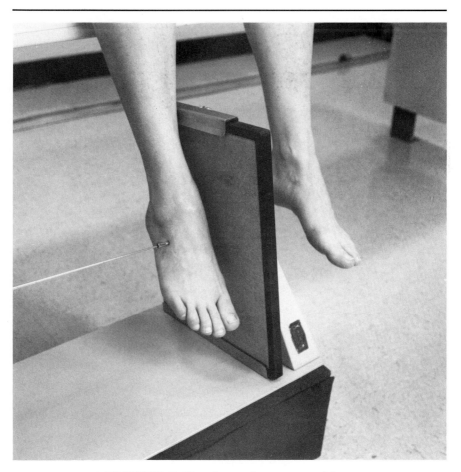

FIGURE 5-10   Lateral stress position.

❖ Ankle

OVERROTATED LATERAL POSITION

Pathology Demonstrated. Degenerative changes involving the posterior portion of the subtalar joint.

The posterior portion of the subtalar joint is often not visualized on routine radiographs of the ankle or foot. A method of overrotating the ankle is useful for demonstrating this portion of the ankle (Figure 5-11).

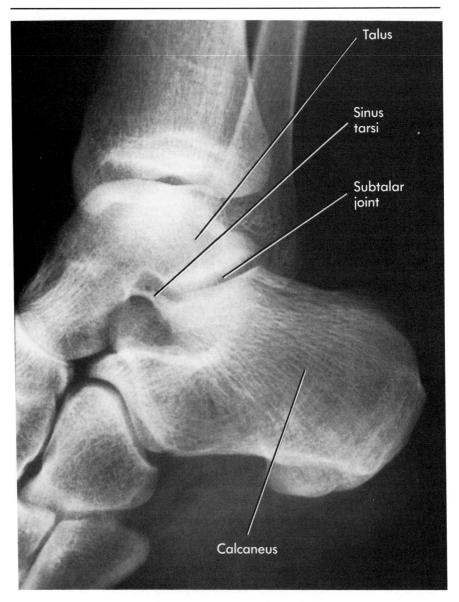

Talus

Sinus tarsi

Subtalar joint

Calcaneus

FIGURE 5-11   Overrotated lateral position.

Patient Position. The patient should be placed in a lateral recumbent position with the affected side down. The lower limb should be fully extended with the ankle on the cassette, which is placed on the radiographic tabletop.

Part Position. The ankle should be placed in a lateral position and should then be externally rotated 10 degrees beyond the lateral position (Figure 5-12).

Central Ray. The central ray should be angled 10 degrees caudad and directed to enter at the talocalcaneal articulation.

Radiograph Evaluation. The posterior portion of the subtalar joint should be demonstrated.

The bony trabeculae of the talus (astragalus) and the calcaneus (os calcis) should be well visualized.

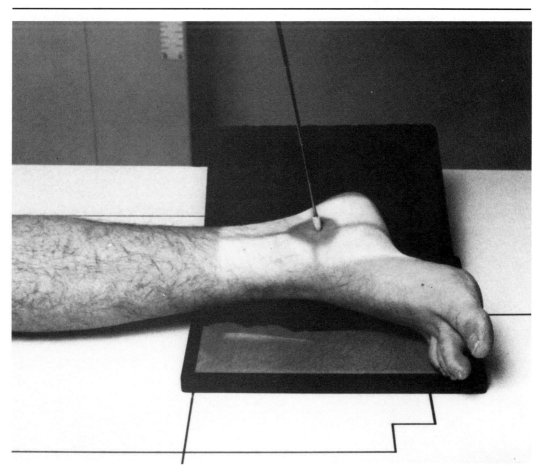

FIGURE 5-12 Overrotated lateral position.

AXIAL OBLIQUE POSITION

Pathology Demonstrated. Talar neck fracture.

The majority of the neck of the talus (astragalus) is often not demonstrated on routine radiographs of the foot. Canale and Kelly[2] indicate a position that is useful for demonstrating this part of the ankle (Figure 5-13).

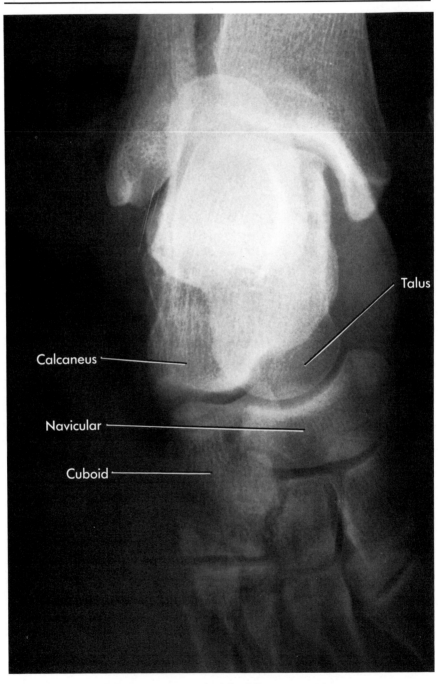

FIGURE 5-13   Axial oblique position.

ANKLE

Patient Position. The patient should be supine on the radiographic table. The affected lower limb should be fully extended with the ankle on the cassette, which is placed on the radiographic tabletop.

Part Position. The affected ankle should be positioned as for a true AP projection. The ankle should then be positioned in maximum plantarflexion (in maximum extension) and should be internally rotated 15 degrees (Figure 5-14).

Central Ray. The central ray should be angled 15 degrees cephalad and directed to enter at the midtarsal region.

Radiograph Evaluation. The majority of the talar neck should be demonstrated and somewhat elongated.

The bony trabeculae of the talus and the articulation of the talus and navicular (scaphoid) should be well visualized.

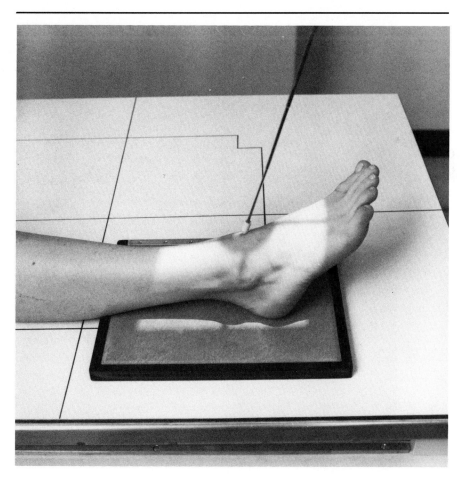

FIGURE 5-14 Axial oblique position.

MEDIAL OBLIQUE POSITION OF THE ANKLE MORTISE

Pathology Demonstrated. Ankle dislocation.

Routine radiographs of the ankle, even the internal oblique, do not fully demonstrate the ankle joint, also known as the ankle mortise. Demonstration of the true ankle mortise is necessary for accurate radiographic interpretation of ankle dislocation. A useful radiographic method for demonstration of the ankle mortise has been described by Wilson[5] and Ballinger[1] (Figure 5-15).

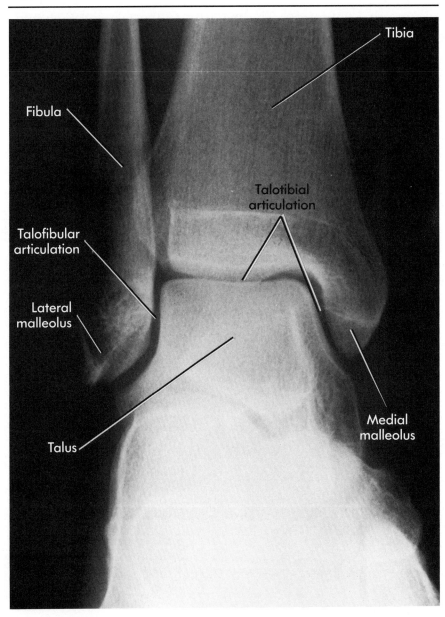

FIGURE 5-15   Medial oblique position of the ankle mortise.

Patient Position. The patient should be supine on the radiographic table. The affected lower limb should be fully extended with the ankle on the cassette, which is placed on the radiographic tabletop.

Part Position. The affected ankle should be positioned as for a true AP projection. The leg and foot should then be internally rotated 10 to 15 degrees according to Wilson,[5] or 15 to 20 degrees according to Ballinger.[1] Regardless of the degree of internal rotation of the ankle the definitive ankle mortise position requires that the internal rotation of the ankle be such that both malleoli are the same distance from the cassette (Figure 5-16).

Central Ray. The central ray should be directed perpendicular to the film to enter at the ankle mortise.

Radiograph Evaluation. The ankle mortise should be demonstrated.

The articulations between both the medial and lateral malleoli and the talus (astragalus) should be well visualized.

The articulation between the tibia and talus should be well visualized.

The bony trabeculae of the tibia, fibula, and talus should be well visualized.

ANKLE

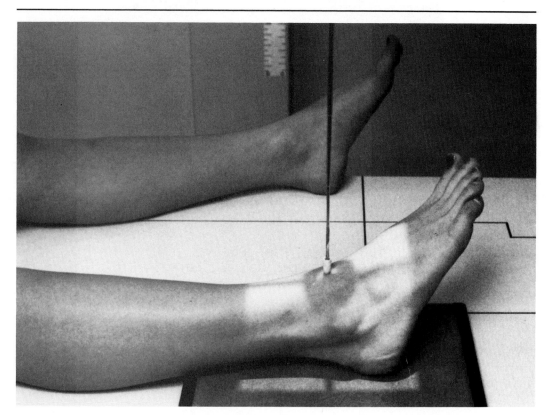

FIGURE 5-16   Medial oblique position of the ankle mortise.

ANKLE

COMPRESSION LATERAL POSITION

Pathology Demonstrated. Subluxation of the talotibial joint.

A method of active compression of the ankle while it is being radiographed in the lateral position is valuable for demonstrating partial dislocation between the talus (astragalus) and the fibula, also known as the drawer sign or talar tilt. Wilson[5] indicates a radiographic method useful for this purpose that places the foot in plantarflexion (extended) (Figure 5-17). Patients who are experiencing a substantial amount of pain should not be examined in this manner without anesthesia.

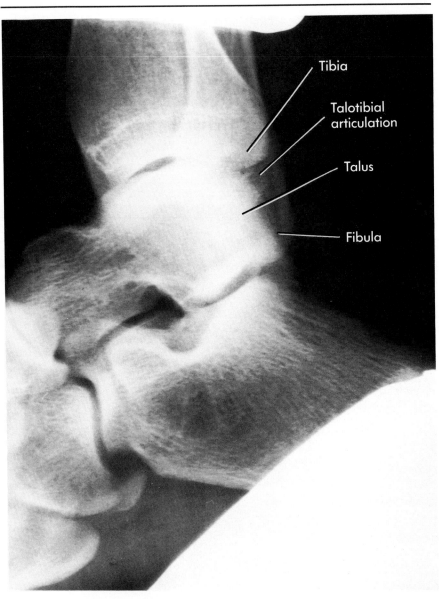

Tibia

Talotibial articulation

Talus

Fibula

FIGURE 5-17   Compression lateral position.

Patient Position. The patient should be placed in a lateral recumbent position on the radiographic table with the affected side down. The affected lower limb should be fully extended with the ankle on the cassette, which is placed on the radiographic tabletop.

Part Position. The affected ankle should be positioned as for a true lateral ankle radiograph. Posterior compression should then be applied against the mid portion of the tibia and fibula while the plantar surface of the foot is held firmly (Figure 5-18). Lead gloves and a lead apron should be worn by the person producing the compression. Wilson[5] indicates that anesthesia and comparison radiographs of the unaffected ankle may be necessary to properly evaluate the extent of injury, if any.

Central Ray. The central ray should be directed perpendicular to the film to pass through the talotibial joint.

Radiograph Evaluation. The ankle should be demonstrated without rotation.
The articulation between the talus and fibula should be well visualized.

ANKLE

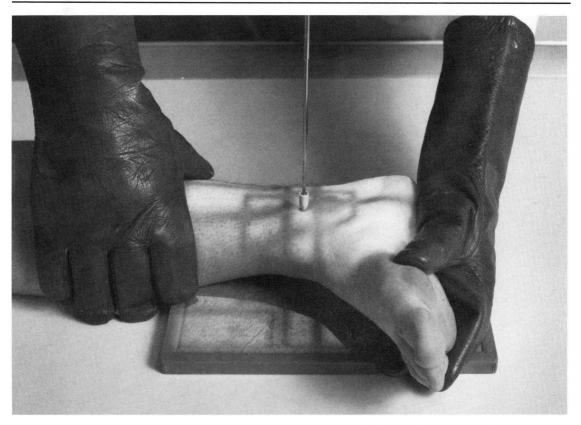

FIGURE 5-18   Compression lateral position.

CHAPTER 5 • REFERENCES

1. Ballinger PW: *Merrill's atlas of radiographic positions and radiologic procedures,* ed 7, vol 1, St. Louis, 1991, Mosby–Year Book.
2. Canale ST, Kelly FB Jr: Fractures of the neck of the talus: long-term evaluation of seventy-one cases, *J Bone Joint Surg* 60A:143, 1978
3. Heckman JD: *Fractures and dislocations of the foot.* In Rockwood CA Jr, Green DP, editors: *Fractures in adults,* ed 2, Philadelphia, 1984, JB Lippincott.
4. McInnes J: *Clark's positioning in radiography,* ed 9, vol 1, St. Louis, 1973, Mosby–Year Book.
5. Wilson FC: *Fractures and dislocations of the ankle.* In Rockwood CA Jr, Green DP, editors: *Fractures in adults,* ed 2, Philadelphia, 1984, JB Lippincott.

The Lower Limb (Patella and Knee)

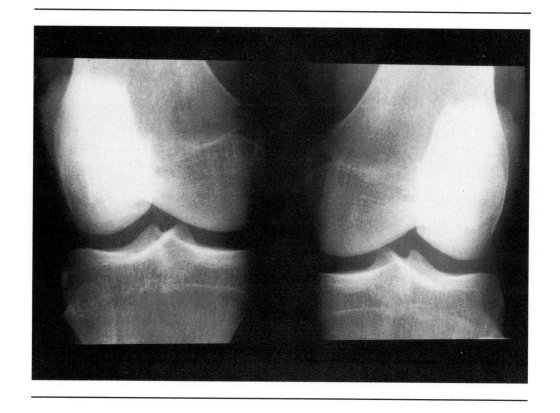

PATELLA

❖ Patella
SITTING TANGENTIAL POSITION

Pathology Demonstrated. Dislocation or chondromalacia of the patella.

Although there are several satisfactory methods for radiographically examining the patellofemoral articulation, many necessitate that the patient assume a position that may be difficult if the patient is in pain or is obese. A method of obtaining a radiograph of the patellofemoral articulation while the patient is sitting (Figure 6-1) is useful in these instances.

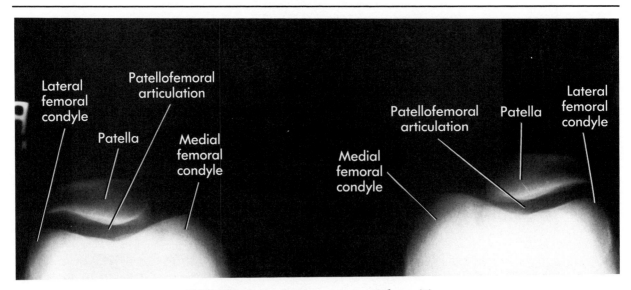

FIGURE 6-1   Sitting tangential position.

Patient Position. The patient should be seated in a stationary chair.

Part Position. The patient should flex the knees as much as is allowed by his or her condition. The cassette should be positioned as close to the patient's knees as possible. This will require that the cassette be built up off the floor using positioning sponges or other available materials. Because of the relatively large object-film distance (object-image distance) the focal-film distance (source-image distance) should be increased to approximately 50 inches (127 cm) or more to decrease radiographic magnification. Both patellofemoral articulations can be examined with one exposure (Figure 6-2), which allows the affected side to be compared with the unaffected side on the same radiograph. Alternatively, the sides can be exposed individually or only the affected side examined.

Central Ray. The central ray should be directed perpendicular to the film. If both articulations are examined on one radiograph, then the central ray should be directed to pass through a point midway between both knees at the level of the patellofemoral articulations. If only one articulation is being examined at a time, then the central ray should be directed to pass through the patellofemoral articulation of interest.

Radiograph Evaluation. One or both patellofemoral articulations should be demonstrated.

One or both patellofemoral articulations should be demonstrated.
The bony trabeculae of the patella (or patellae) should be well visualized.
One or both patellofemoral articulations should be well visualized.

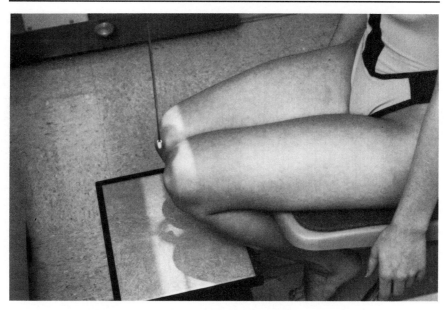

FIGURE 6-2   Sitting tangential position.

FLEXION LATERAL POSITION

Pathology Demonstrated. Patella alta.

Larson and Jones[2] indicate that a lateral with the knee positioned in a 90-degree flexion position (Figure 6-3) should be conducted as part of a patella survey because routine radiographs of the knee are of little value in assessing or diagnosing patella alta. Patella alta, also referred to as a high-riding patella, is defined as a patella that is intersected by a line extending down the anterior aspect of the shaft of the femur. Normally this line should pass over the patella without intersecting it.

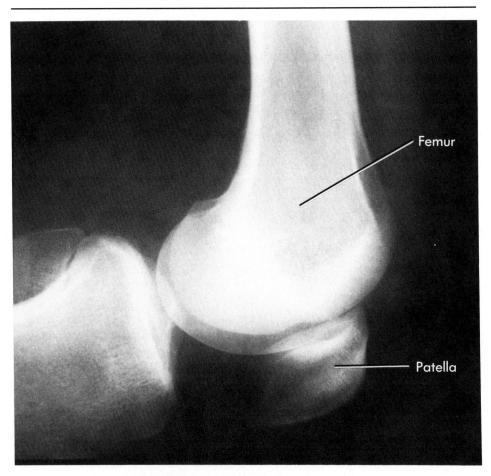

FIGURE 6-3   Flexion lateral position.

Patient Position. The patient should be positioned in a lateral recumbent position on the affected side with the knee on the cassette, which is placed on the radiographic tabletop. The cassette may instead be placed in the Bucky tray.

Part Position. The affected knee should be flexed 90 degrees (Figure 6-4).

Central Ray. The central ray should be angled 5 degrees cephalad and directed to pass through the patellofemoral articulation.

Radiograph Evaluation. The patella and distal femur should be demonstrated without rotation.

The knee should be flexed 90 degrees.

PATELLA

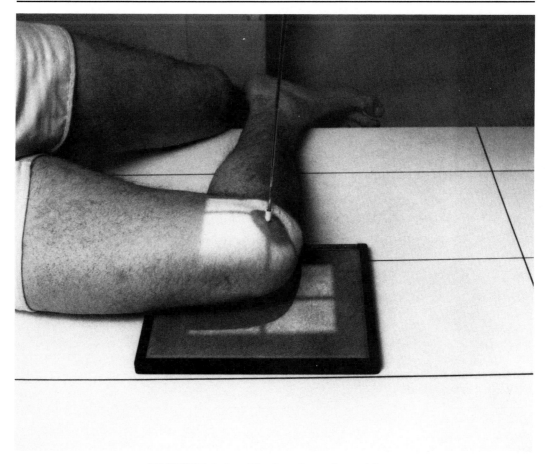

FIGURE 6-4   Flexion lateral position.

❖ Knee

WEIGHT-BEARING PA AXIAL POSITION

Pathology Demonstrated. Degenerative arthritis of the knee joints.

To adequately demonstrate degenerative arthritis of the knee joints the radiograph must give complete visual access to the joint spaces. Routine radiographs of the knee do not generally offer this view. A weight-bearing PA axial position of the knee joints performed bilaterally (Figure 6-5) is useful for this purpose.

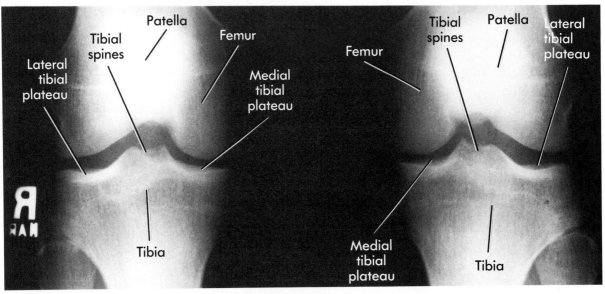

FIGURE 6-5 Weight-bearing PA axial position.

Patient Position. The patient should be standing and facing the upright film-holding device, which holds the cassette.

Part Position. The patient's knees should be positioned close to each other and flexed 20 degrees (Figure 6-6).

Central Ray. The central ray should be angled 10 degrees caudad and directed to pass midway between both knees at the level of the knee joints.

Radiograph Evaluation. Both knee joints should be demonstrated.
 The knee joints should be well visualized.
 The bony trabeculae of the femora and tibiae should be well visualized.

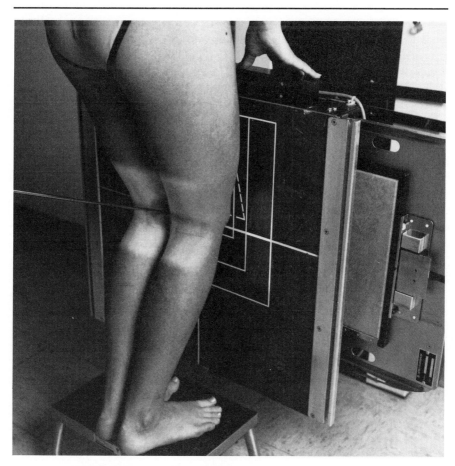

FIGURE 6-6   Weight-bearing PA axial position.

KNEE

AP STRESS PROJECTIONS

Pathology Demonstrated. Medial collateral ligament and lateral ligament insufficiency.

To assess injury to the medial collateral and lateral collateral ligaments of the knee as indicated by either medial or lateral knee joint widening, respectively, AP stress projections of the knee must be produced. Patients who are experiencing a substantial amount of pain should not be examined in this manner without anesthesia; this method is valuable for patients who are able to cooperate. For these radiographs the patient must apply either medial or lateral stress with the knees. Each radiograph is named for the direction of stress as applied by the patient. For the AP medial stress projection of the knees the knees are stressed by the patient in a medial direction (Figure 6-7) to assess the sufficiency of the medial collateral ligament. For the AP lateral stress projection of the knees the knees are stressed by the patient in a lateral direction (Figure 6-8) to assess the sufficiency of the lateral collateral ligament.

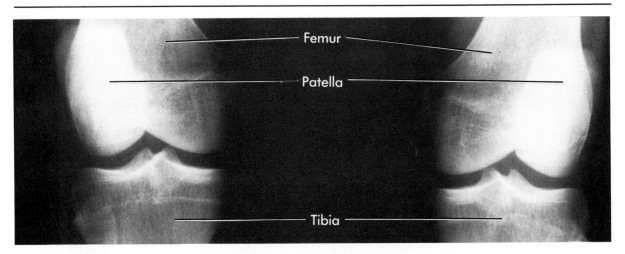

FIGURE 6-7   AP stress projection.

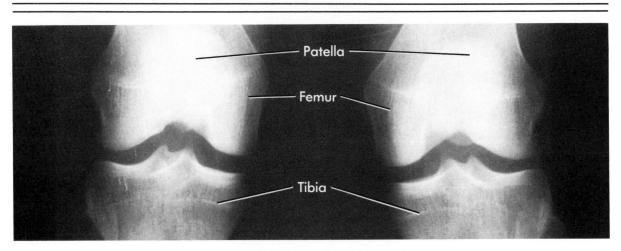

FIGURE 6-8   AP stress projection.

Patient Position. For both the AP medial and AP lateral stress projections of the knee the patient should be positioned in a supine recumbent position on the radiographic table.

Part Position. For the AP medial stress projection the knees should be positioned in a true AP position and in contact with the cassette, which is placed on the radiographic tabletop. The cassette may instead be placed in the Bucky tray. The patient is asked to stress both knees in a medial direction. Counter stress is applied by another person who is standing at the end of the radiographic table and is providing resistance in a lateral direction (Figure 6-9). The exposure should be made while the patient is stressing the knees. The person who is providing counter stress against the patient should wear lead gloves and a lead apron.

For the AP lateral stress projection the knees should be positioned in a true AP position and in contact with the cassette, which is placed on the radiographic tabletop. The cassette may instead be placed in the Bucky tray. The patient is asked to stress both knees in a lateral direction. Counter stress is applied by another person who is standing at the end of the radiographic table and is providing resistance in a medial direction (Figure 6-10). The exposure should be made while the patient is stressing the knees. Care should be taken to use a film that is large enough to image both knees with a single exposure. The person who is providing counter stress against the patient should wear lead gloves and a lead apron.

Central Ray. For both radiographs the central ray should be angled 5 to 7 degrees cephalad and directed to pass midway between both knees at the level of the knee joints.

Radiograph Evaluation. Both knees should be demonstrated with both medial and lateral stress.

The joint spaces of both knees should be well visualized.

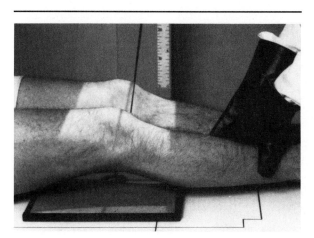

FIGURE 6-9 AP stress projection.

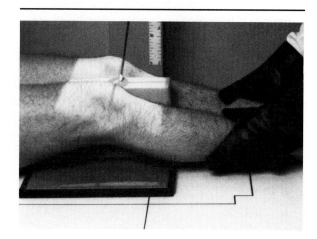

FIGURE 6-10 AP stress projection.

LATERAL STRESS POSITION

Pathology Demonstrated. Posterior cruciate ligament insufficiency.

To assess injury to the posterior cruciate ligament Muller[3] indicates that the knee must be stressed and radiographed in the lateral position (Figure 6-11). Patients who are experiencing a substantial amount of pain should not be examined in this manner without anesthesia. Posterior cruciate ligament insufficiency is indicated by posterior displacement of the lateral tibial plateau in relation to the lateral femoral condyle.

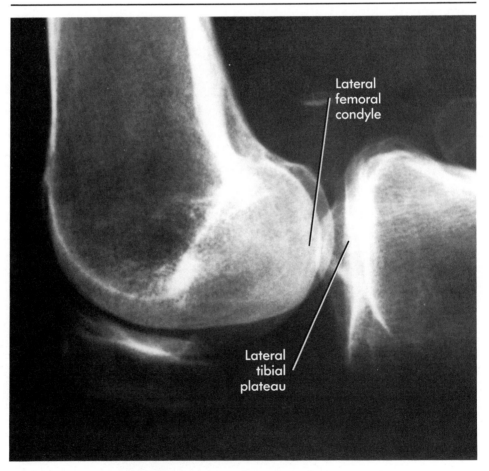

Lateral
femoral
condyle

Lateral
tibial
plateau

FIGURE 6-11   Lateral stress position.

Patient Position. The patient should be positioned in a lateral recumbent position on the radiographic table with the affected side down. The knee should be on the cassette, which is placed on the radiographic tabletop. The cassette may instead be placed in the Bucky tray.

Part Position. The affected knee should be positioned in a lateral position and flexed 90 degrees (Figure 6-12). Posterior stress should be applied to the proximal tibia and fibula by another person. The same person should also provide resistance in an anterior direction to the distal tibia and fibula. The person who is providing resistance should wear lead gloves and a lead apron.

Central Ray. The central ray should be angled 5 degrees cephalad and directed to pass through the knee joint.

Radiograph Evaluation. The knee should be demonstrated without rotation.
   The knee should be flexed 90 degrees.
   The knee joint should be well visualized.

KNEE

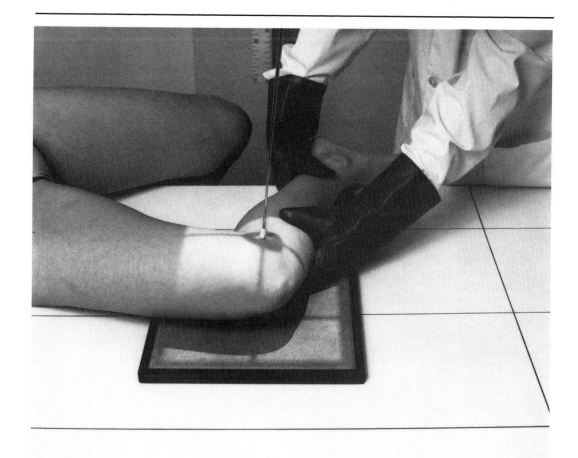

FIGURE 6-12   Lateral stress position.

EXTENSION LATERAL POSITION

Pathology Demonstrated. Avulsion fracture of the intercondylar eminences in children.

A routine lateral position of the knee may not show an avulsion fracture of the intercondylar eminences in children. Instead, Roberts[4] indicates that a lateral knee in full extension (Figure 6-13) is valuable for demonstrating the avulsed fracture fragment near the distal end of the femur.

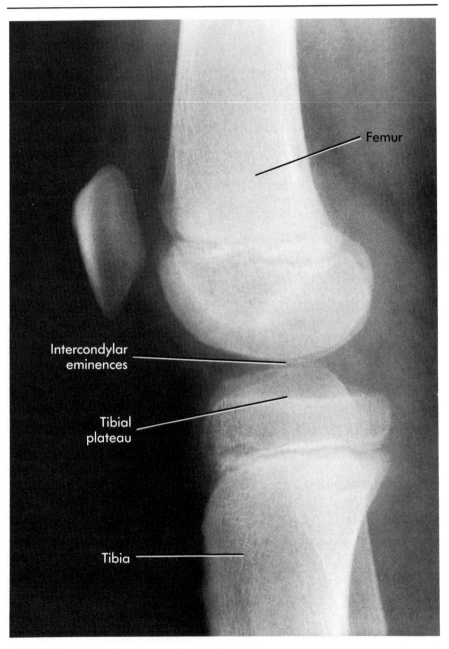

FIGURE 6-13   Extension lateral position.

Patient Position. The patient should be positioned in a lateral recumbent position on the radiographic table with the affected side down. The knee should be on the cassette, which is placed on the radiographic tabletop. The cassette may instead be placed in the Bucky tray.

Part Position. The affected knee should be placed in a lateral position and fully extended (Figure 6-14).

Central Ray. The central ray should be angled 5 degrees cephalad and directed to pass through the knee joint.

Radiograph Evaluation. The knee should be demonstrated with no rotation and fully extended.

The knee joint and bony trabeculae of the femur and tibia should be well visualized.

KNEE

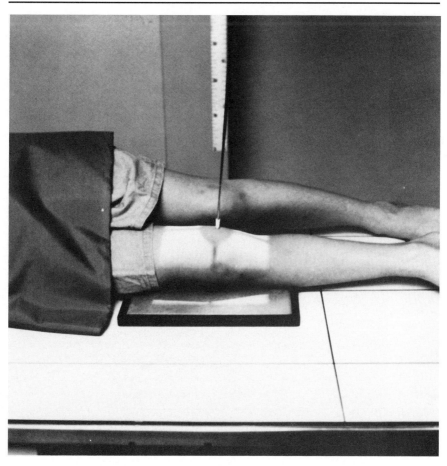

FIGURE 6-14　Extension lateral position.

KNEE

PA FEMORAL EPIPHYSEAL PROJECTION

Pathology Demonstrated. Posterior distal femoral growth arrest in children.

In children the central ray on routine AP and PA projections of the knee does not pass directly through the epiphyseal space of the distal femur. Bright[1] indicates that a PA projection of the flexed knee (Figure 6-15) allows the central ray to pass directly through the distal femoral epiphyseal space and is useful for demonstrating growth arrest in this area.

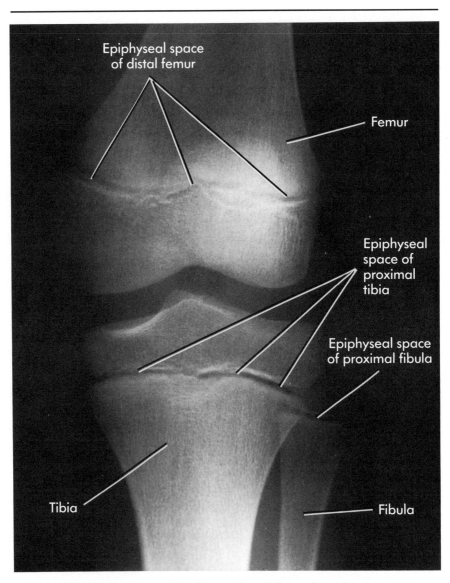

Epiphyseal space
of distal femur

Femur

Epiphyseal
space of
proximal
tibia

Epiphyseal space
of proximal fibula

Tibia

Fibula

FIGURE 6-15   PA femoral epiphyseal projection.

Patient Position. The patient should be positioned in a prone recumbent position on the radiographic table. The affected knee should be on the cassette, which is placed on the radiographic tabletop. The cassette may instead be placed in the Bucky tray.

Part Position. The patient's trunk should be elevated so that the affected knee is flexed 30 to 45 degrees (Figure 6-16). Elevation of the patient's trunk can be accomplished by having the patient lie over a step stool that is made comfortable with the aid of a pillow. Other means of elevation can be used.

Central Ray. The central ray should be directed perpendicular to the film and directed to enter superior to the knee joint and pass through the distal femoral epiphyseal space.

Radiograph Evaluation. The knee should be demonstrated with no rotation and with 30 to 45 degrees of flexion.

The distal femoral epiphyseal space should be well visualized.

KNEE

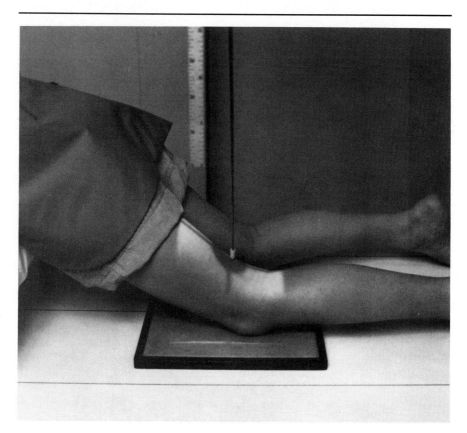

FIGURE 6-16 PA femoral epiphyseal projection.

LATERAL FEMORAL EPIPHYSEAL POSITION

Pathology Demonstrated. Lateral distal femoral growth arrest in children.

In children the central ray on routine lateral positions of the knee does not pass directly through the epiphyseal space of the distal femur. Bright[1] indicates that a lateral position of the knee with the shaft of the femur elevated away from the film (Figure 6-17) allows the central ray to pass directly through the distal femoral epiphyseal space and is useful for demonstrating growth arrest in this area.

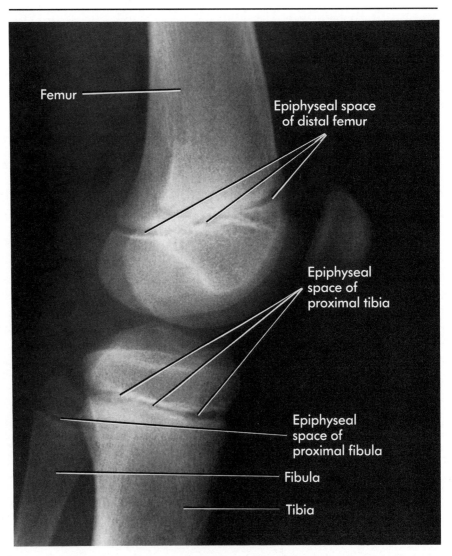

FIGURE 6-17 Lateral femoral epiphyseal position.

Patient Position. The patient should be positioned in a lateral recumbent position on the radiographic table with the unaffected side down. The cassette, which is placed on the radiographic tabletop, should be placed directly under the affected knee and be in contact with only the proximal tibia and fibula. The cassette may instead be placed in the Bucky tray.

Part Position. The affected lower limb should be extended, slightly flexed, and positioned posterior to the unaffected lower limb (Figure 6-18).

Central Ray. The central ray should be directed perpendicular to the film to enter superior to the knee joint and pass directly through the distal femoral epiphyseal space.

Radiograph Evaluation. The knee should be demonstrated in a lateral position with slight flexion.
    The distal femoral epiphyseal space should be well visualized.

KNEE

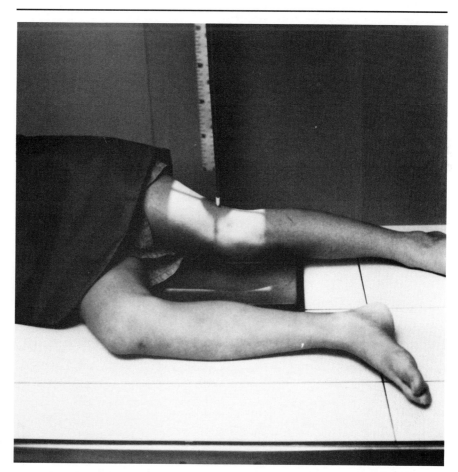

FIGURE 6-18   Lateral femoral epiphyseal position.

CHAPTER 6 • REFERENCES

1. Bright RW: *Physeal injuries.* In Rockwood CA Jr, Wilkins KE, King RE, editors: *Fractures in children,* Philadelphia, 1984, JB Lippincott.
2. Larson RL, Jones DC: *Dislocations and ligamentous injuries of the knee.* In Rockwood CA Jr, Green DP, editors: *Fractures in adults,* ed 2, Philadelphia, 1984, JB Lippincott.
3. Muller ME: *Intertrochanteric osteotomies.* In Evarts CM, editor: *Surgery of the musculoskeletal system,* vol 3, New York, 1983, Churchill Livingstone.
4. Roberts JM: *Fractures and dislocations of the knee.* In Rockwood CA Jr, Wilkins KE, King RE, editors: *Fractures in children,* Philadelphia, 1984, JB Lippincott.

CHAPTER
7

The Hip, Pelvis, and Spine

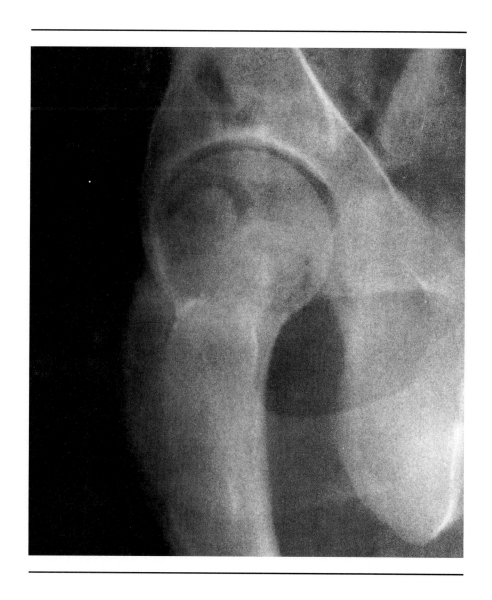

❖ Hip

ABDUCTION AND ADDUCTION AP PROJECTIONS

Pathology Demonstrated. Osteoarthritis of the hip.

Routine radiographs of the hip are capable of demonstrating osteoarthritis of the hip; however, Muller[6] indicates that two range-of-motion radiographs of the hip, an AP abduction projection (Figure 7-1) and an AP adduction projection (Figure 7-2), are valuable for further assessment.

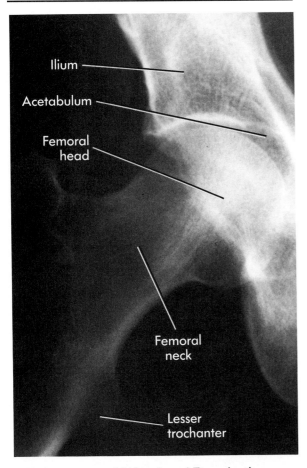

FIGURE 7-1 Abduction AP projection.

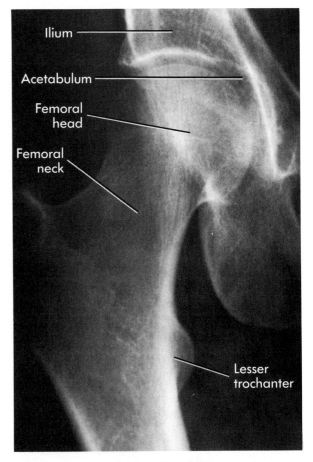

FIGURE 7-2 Adduction AP projection.

Patient Position. The patient should be placed in a supine position on the radiographic table with the cassette placed in the Bucky tray.

Part Position. For the AP abduction projection of the hip the affected hip, tube, and film should first be aligned to one another. The affected lower limb should then be abducted so that the affected foot rests off of the radiographic table (Figure 7-3).

For the AP adduction projection of the affected hip the affected lower limb should be adducted as much as possible. The unaffected lower limb should then be flexed and crossed over the affected lower limb. The plantar surface of the unaffected foot should be positioned flat on the radiographic tabletop (Figure 7-4).

Central Ray. The central ray for both radiographs should be directed perpendicular to the film to pass through the femoral neck.

Radiograph Evaluation. The affected hip should be demonstrated in both abduction and adduction.

The bony trabeculae of the proximal femur and acetabulum should be well visualized.

The hip joint should be well visualized.

HIP

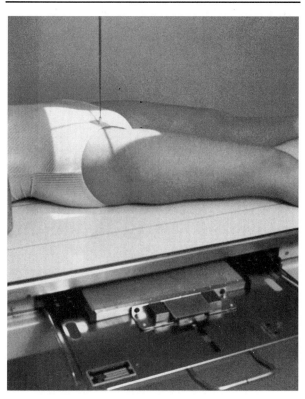

FIGURE 7-3 Abduction AP projection.

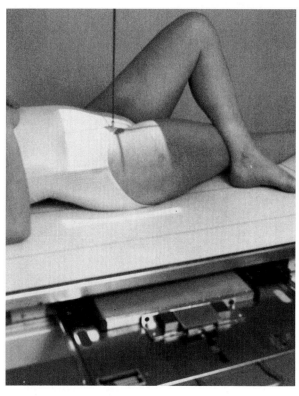

FIGURE 7-4 Adduction AP projection.

WEIGHT-BEARING ACETABULAR OBLIQUE POSITIONS

Pathology Demonstrated. Hip joint narrowing.

Routine radiographs of the hip joint may demonstrate narrowing of the space between the femoral head and the acetabulum but do not demonstrate whether the narrowing occurs in the anterior or posterior portion of the acetabulum. By producing a radiograph of the weight-bearing hip with the patient positioned in an anterior oblique position (Figure 7-5), hip joint narrowing of the anterior portion of the acetabulum can be assessed. By producing a radiograph of the weight-bearing hip with the patient positioned in a posterior oblique position (Figure 7-6), hip joint narrowing of the posterior portion of the acetabulum can be assessed.

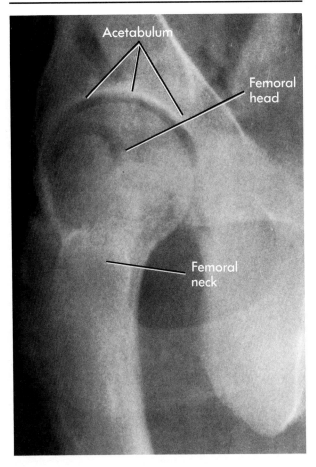

FIGURE 7-5 Weight-bearing acetabular oblique position (RAO).

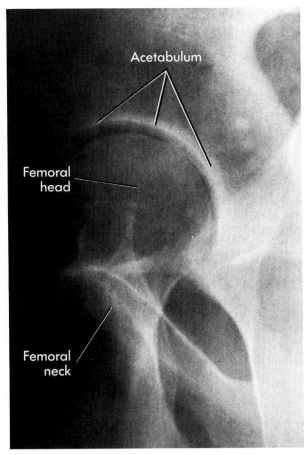

FIGURE 7-6 Weight-bearing acetabular oblique position (RPO).

Patient Position. The patient should be standing with the affected hip against the upright film-holding device, which holds the cassette. The patient's arms should be folded across the chest.

Part Position. To demonstrate the right hip the patient should be positioned in a 20-degree RAO (Figure 7-7) for one radiograph and in a 20-degree RPO (Figure 7-8) for the next radiograph. The left hip can be demonstrated with a 20-degree LAO and LPO.

Central Ray. The central ray should be directed perpendicular to the film to pass through the affected hip.

Radiograph Evaluation. The anterior portion of the acetabulum should be demonstrated on the anterior oblique, and the posterior portion of the acetabulum should be demonstrated on the posterior oblique.

The bony trabeculae of the acetabulum should be well visualized.

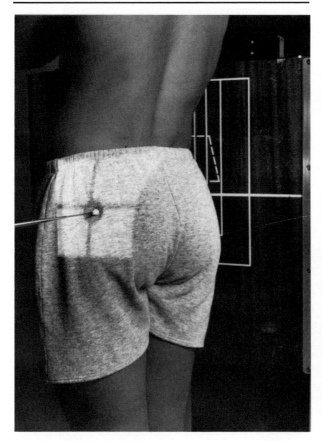

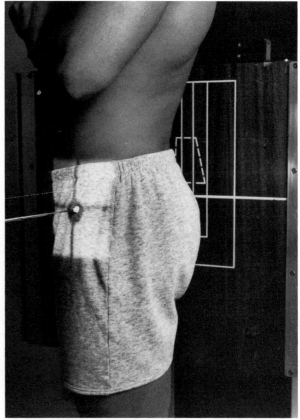

FIGURE 7-7 Weight-bearing acetabular oblique position (RAO).

FIGURE 7-8 Weight-bearing acetabular oblique position (RPO).

SITTING AP PROJECTION

Pathology Demonstrated. Hip fracture.

For some patients with a possible hip fracture it is more comfortable to sit in a semiupright position than to be supine. McInnes[5] indicates that the routine AP projection (Figure 7-9) can still be accomplished with a patient who prefers to be examined in a sitting position. This method is not recommended, however, for obese patients with large abdomens.

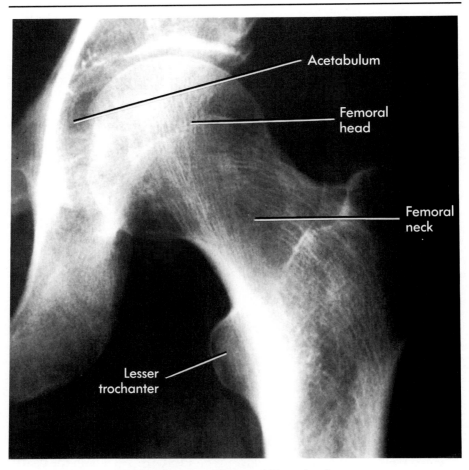

FIGURE 7-9 Sitting AP projection.

Patient Position. The patient should be positioned in a semiupright sitting position either on a patient cart or on the radiographic table. Some patients will be able to support themselves in this position and some will need additional support. If additional support is needed it is recommended that the patient be examined on a cart of which one end may be elevated.

Part Position. If possible, the legs should be abducted several inches from each other. The grid and cassette should be placed on the radiographic tabletop or the patient cart, directly under and centered to the affected hip (Figure 7-10). If the radiographic table is used, it may be possible to use the Bucky device in the table if the patient can be centered to it.

Central Ray. The central ray should be directed perpendicular to the film to pass through the femoral neck.

Radiograph Evaluation. The acetabulum, hip joint, and proximal femur should be demonstrated.

The bony trabeculae of the acetabulum and proximal femur should be well visualized.

The hip joint should be well visualized.

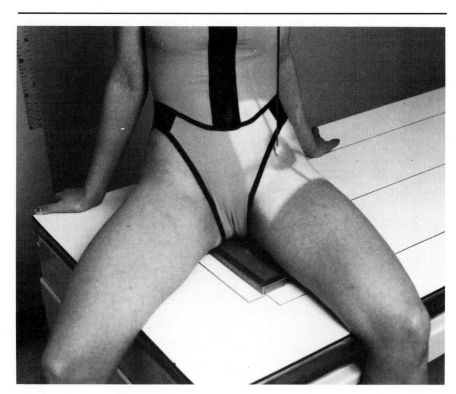

FIGURE 7-10 Sitting AP projection.

SITTING LATERAL POSITION

Pathology Demonstrated. Hip fracture.

For some patients with a possible hip fracture it is more comfortable to sit in a semiupright position than to be supine. McInnes[5] indicates that a lateral position radiograph (Figure 7-11) can still be obtained with a patient who prefers to be examined in a sitting position.

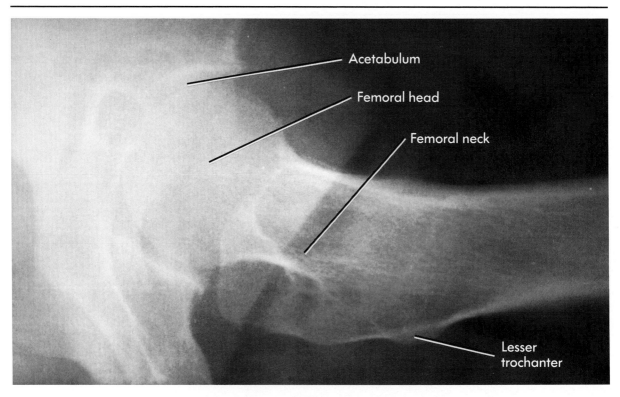

FIGURE 7-11   Sitting lateral position.

Patient Position. The patient should be positioned in a semiupright sitting position either on a patient cart or on the radiographic table. The unaffected leg should be allowed to dangle over the side. If the radiographic table is being used, it is also easier to allow the patient to dangle the affected leg over the side of the table. Some patients will be able to support themselves in this position and some will need additional support. If additional support is needed, it is recommended that the patient be examined on a cart of which one end can be elevated.

Part Position. The legs should be abducted several inches from each other. The grid and cassette should be positioned vertically and centered to and in contact with the lateral surface of the affected hip (Figure 7-12).

Central Ray. The central ray should be directed perpendicular to the film to pass through the femoral neck.

Radiograph Evaluation. The acetabulum, hip joint, and proximal femur should be demonstrated.

The bony trabeculae of the acetabulum and proximal femur should be well visualized.

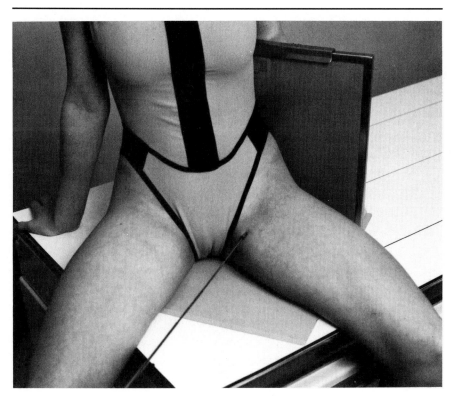

FIGURE 7-12 Sitting lateral position.

❖ Pelvis

RPO OR LPO (AP OBLIQUE) POSITION

Pathology Demonstrated. Acetabular fracture.

Fractures of the acetabulum are easily demonstrated by the routine AP projection of the pelvis or hip. However, the AP projection makes it difficult to localize the site of the fracture and the position of fracture fragments. Fisk[1] indicates that an oblique of the hip rotated slightly from the lateral (Figure 7-13) is valuable for better assessing acetabular fractures and the position of fracture fragments.

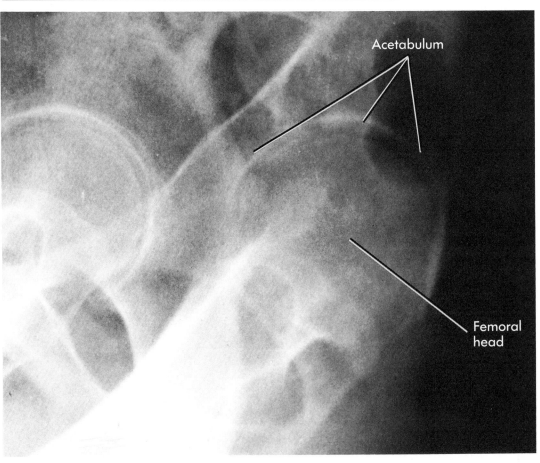

FIGURE 7-13   RPO (AP oblique) position.

Patient Position. The patient should be placed in a lateral recumbent position on the radiographic table with the unaffected side down. The cassette should be placed in the Bucky tray.

Part Position. From the lateral position the patient should be rolled posteriorly 30 degrees to obtain a 60-degree posterior oblique. To examine the left hip the right hip should be closer to the film and the patient rolled posteriorly 30 degrees to obtain a 60-degree RPO (Figure 7-14). To examine the right hip the left hip should be closer to the film and the patient rolled posteriorly 30 degrees to obtain a 60-degree LPO.

Central Ray. The central ray should be directed perpendicular to the film to pass through the femoral head of the affected hip.

Radiograph Evaluation. The acetabulum should be demonstrated.

The affected acetabulum should be magnified in comparison with the unaffected hip.

The bony trabeculae of the affected acetabulum should be well visualized.

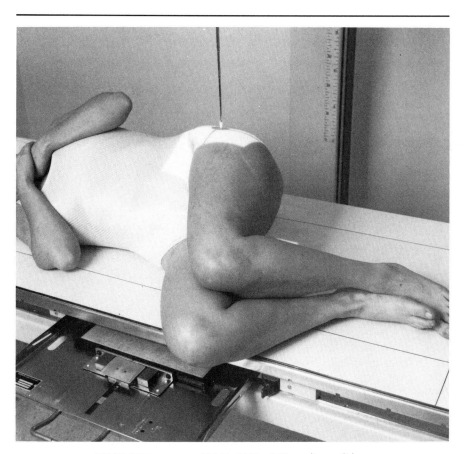

FIGURE 7-14   RPO (AP oblique) position.

FLEXION RPO OR LPO (AP OBLIQUE) POSITION

Pathology Demonstrated. Acetabular fracture.

Another method of demonstrating acetabular fractures exists. Kane[3] indicates that an oblique of the hip rotated slightly from the lateral and with the femora positioned at a 90-degree angle to the pelvis (Figure 7-15) is valuable for better assessing acetabular fractures and the position of fracture fragments.

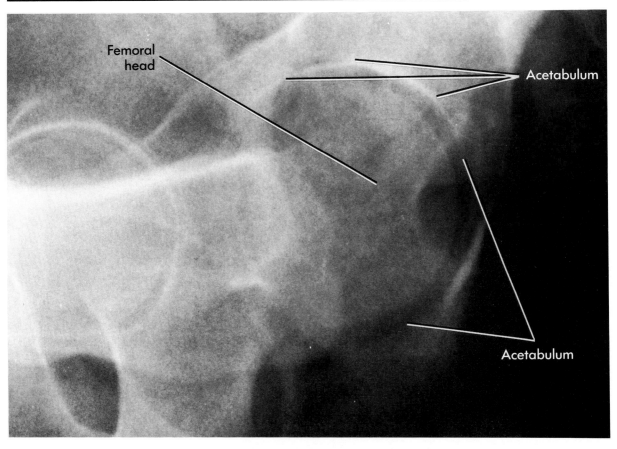

FIGURE 7-15   Flexion RPO (AP oblique) position.

Patient Position. The patient should be placed in a lateral recumbent position on the radiographic table with the unaffected side down. The cassette should be placed in the Bucky tray.

Part Position. From the lateral position the patient should be rolled posteriorly 30 degrees to obtain a 60-degree posterior oblique. The femora should be flexed toward the pelvis to form a 90-degree angle with the pelvis. To examine the left hip the right hip should be the closer to the film and the patient rolled posteriorly 30 degrees to obtain a 60-degree RPO (Figure 7-16). To examine the right hip the left hip should be closer to the film and the patient rolled posteriorly 30 degrees to obtain a 60-degree LPO.

Central Ray. The central ray should be directed perpendicular to the film to pass through the femoral head of the affected hip.

Radiograph Evaluation. The acetabulum should be demonstrated with the femora positioned at a 90-degree angle to the pelvis.

The affected acetabulum should be magnified in comparison with the unaffected hip.

The bony trabeculae of the affected acetabulum should be well visualized.

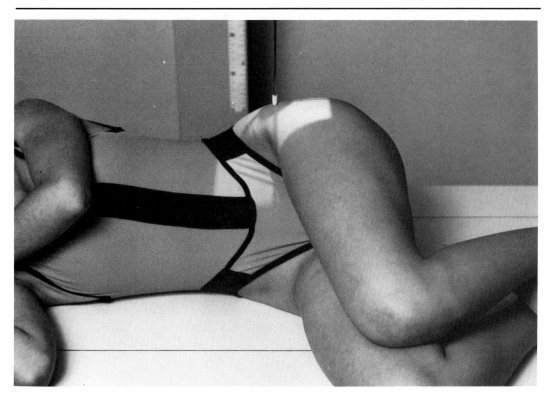

FIGURE 7-16 Flexion RPO (AP oblique) position.

RPO AND LPO POSITIONS: JUDET METHOD

Pathology Demonstrated. Acetabular fracture.

A final method for better demonstrating acetabular fractures also involves an oblique position of the patient. Judet, Judet, and Letournel[2] indicate that a 45-degree posterior oblique of the hip (Figure 7-17) is valuable for assessing fractures of the acetabulum.

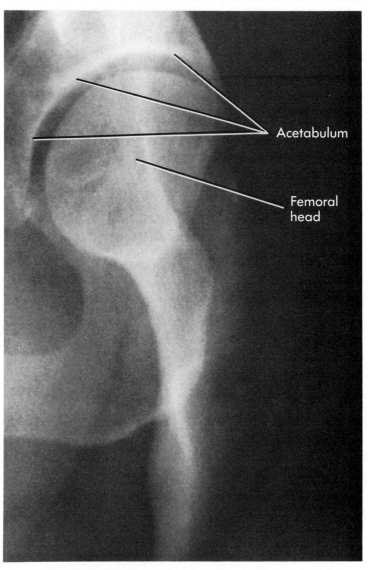

FIGURE 7-17   RPO position: Judet method.

Patient Position. The patient should be placed in a supine position on the radiographic table. The cassette should be placed in the Bucky tray.

Part Position. If the right hip is affected, the patient should be positioned in a 45-degree LPO with both lower limbs extended. If the left hip is affected, the patient should be positioned in a 45-degree RPO with both lower limbs extended (Figure 7-18).

Central Ray. The central ray should be directed perpendicular to the film to pass through the femoral head of the hip of interest.

Radiograph Evaluation. The acetabulum should be demonstrated.
   The bony trabeculae of the acetabulum should be well visualized.

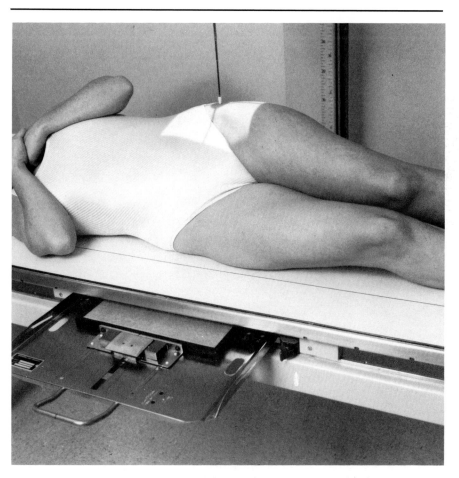

FIGURE 7-18   RPO position: Judet method.

❖ Thoracolumbar Spine

AP PROJECTION

Pathology Demonstrated. Vertebral body fractures.

Kaufer and Kling[4] indicate that over 50% of all vertebral body fractures occur between and including the twelfth thoracic (T12) vertebra and the second lumbar (L2) vertebra. Additionally, 40% of all spinal cord injuries occur between and including T12 and the first lumbar vertebra (L1). Most protocols for spinal radiography, however, divide the spinal column into its three divisions, cervical, thoracic, and lumbar, for radiographic examination. Kaufer and Kling indicate that it is valuable to use a thoracolumbar spine routine in which an AP projection radiograph (Figure 7-19) and a lateral position radiograph (see p. 150) are produced for better assessment of spinal column injury to the inferior thoracic and superior lumbar regions of the spine.

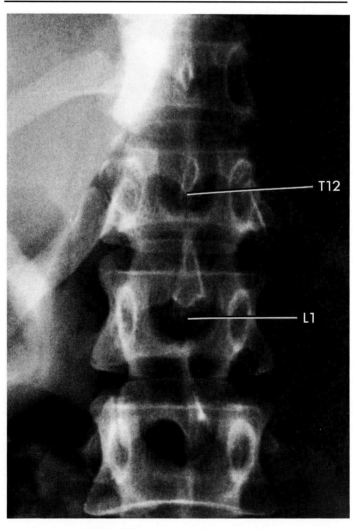

FIGURE 7-19   AP projection.

Patient Position. For the AP projection the patient should be placed in a supine position on the radiographic table with the upper limbs positioned away from the region of the thoracolumbar spine. The cassette should be placed in the Bucky tray.

Part Position. The lower limbs should be flexed somewhat toward the abdomen while the feet remain flat on the radiographic tabletop (Figure 7-20) to bring the spine somewhat closer to the radiographic table.

Central Ray. The central ray should be directed perpendicular to the film to enter at a point approximately halfway between the xiphoid process (ensiform cartilage) and the crest of the ilium (iliac crest).

Radiograph Evaluation. The vertebral column from at least T12 through L2 should be demonstrated without rotation.

The bony trabeculae of all vertebrae demonstrated should be well visualized.
The spine should appear straight.

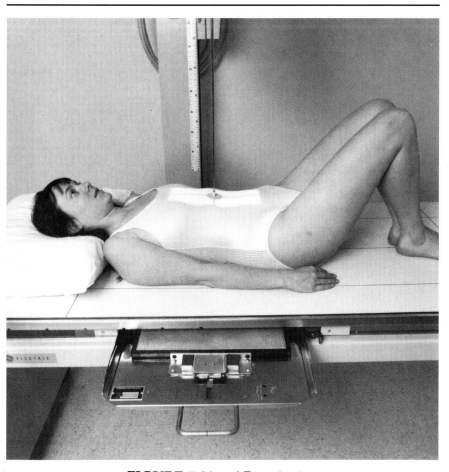

FIGURE 7-20 AP projection.

THORACOLUMBAR SPINE

LATERAL POSITION

Pathology Demonstrated. Vertebral body fractures.

See Thoracolumbar Spine, AP Projection, Pathology Demonstrated, p. 148. Like the AP projection radiograph, the lateral position radiograph (Figure 7-21) is useful for assessing this frequently traumatized region of the spinal column.

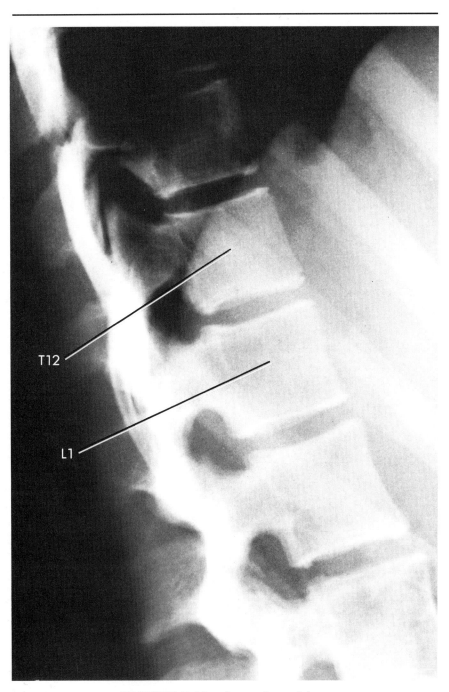

T12

L1

FIGURE 7-21   Lateral position.

Patient Position. For the lateral position the patient should be placed in a left lateral recumbent position on the radiographic table with the upper limbs positioned away from the region of the thoracolumbar spine. The cassette should be placed in the Bucky tray.

Part Position. The lower limbs should be positioned on top of each other and flexed somewhat toward the abdomen (Figure 7-22) to stabilize the patient's position. To keep the spine parallel to the film it may be necessary to use a positioning sponge; it should be placed superior to the crest of the ilium. Scatter radiation exposure to the film used to produce the lateral position radiograph should be kept to a minimum by using a strip of lead. The lead should be positioned behind the patient and on top of the radiographic tabletop.

Central Ray. The central ray should be directed perpendicular to the film to enter the midaxillary plane at a point approximately halfway between the xiphoid process and the crest of the ilium.

Radiograph Evaluation. The vertebral column from at least T12 through L2 should be demonstrated without rotation.

The bony trabeculae of all vertebrae demonstrated should be well visualized.
The intervertebral disk spaces should be well visualized.

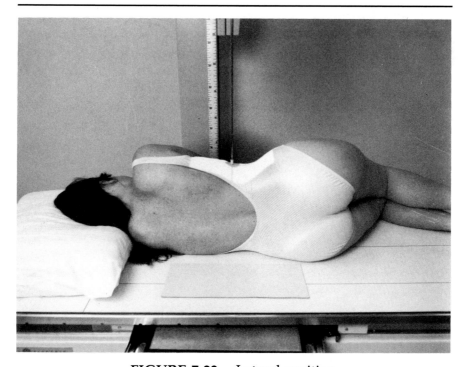

FIGURE 7-22 Lateral position.

❖ Lumbar Spine
BILATERAL L5 THROUGH S1 LATERAL POSITIONS

Pathology Demonstrated. Lumbar scoliosis.

Routine radiographs of the lumbar spine are valuable for assessing scoliosis of the lumbar spine. However, the fifth lumbar (L5) through the first sacral (S1) intervertebral disk space is often not fully visible on the AP projection or lateral position radiograph. Additionally, a single lateral of the L5 through S1 disk space may be of little value. Bilateral laterals of the L5 through S1 disk space (Figures 7-23 and 7-24) are valuable for accurately determining disk-space height in cases of lumbar scoliosis.

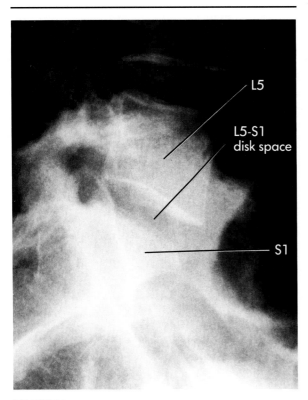

FIGURE 7-23 Left lateral position, L5 through S1.

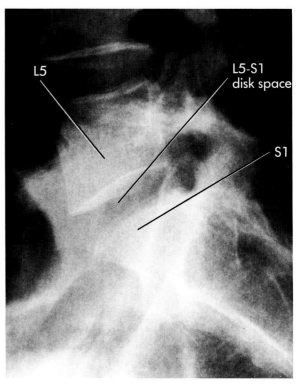

FIGURE 7-24 Right lateral position, L5 through S1.

Patient Position. The patient should be placed in a lateral recumbent position on the radiographic table with the upper limbs positioned away from the region of the L5 through S1 disk space. The cassette should be placed in the Bucky tray. It does not matter which lateral position is achieved first, the right or the left. The method of producing a diagnostic lateral position is the same for both lateral positions.

Part Position. To produce a lateral position of the L5 through S1 disk space the lower limbs should be positioned on top of each other and flexed somewhat toward the abdomen (Figures 7-25 and 7-26) to stabilize the patient's position. To keep the spine parallel to the film it may be necessary to use a positioning sponge; it should be placed superior to the crest of the ilium.

Central Ray. The central ray should be directed 5 to 8 degrees caudad, depending on patient body habitus, to pass through the L5 through S1 disk space. After producing one lateral position radiograph the patient should be positioned for the opposite lateral position.

Radiograph Evaluation. The L5 through S1 disk space should be demonstrated on both radiographs without rotation.

    The L5 through S1 disk space should be well visualized on both radiographs.

LUMBAR SPINE

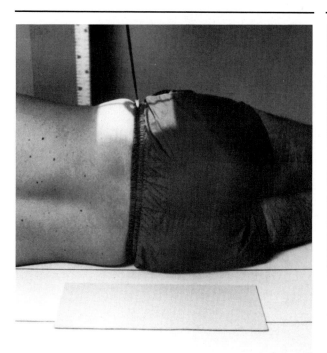

FIGURE 7-25   Left lateral position, L5 through S1.

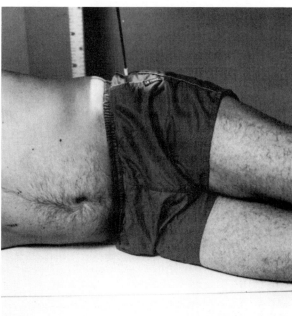

FIGURE 7-26   Right lateral position, L5 through S1.

CHAPTER 7 • REFERENCES

1. Fisk C: Acetabular fractures–where? *Radiol Technol* 35:330, 1964.
2. Judet R, Judet J, Letournel E: Fractures of the acetabulum: classification and surgical approaches for open reduction, *J Bone Joint Surg* 46A:1615, 1964.
3. Kane WJ: *Fractures of the pelvis.* In Rockwood CA Jr, Green DP, editors: *Fractures in adults,* ed 2, Philadelphia, 1984, JB Lippincott.
4. Kaufer H, Kling TF: *The thoracolumbar spine.* In Rockwood CA Jr, Green DP, editors: *Fractures in adults,* ed 2, Philadelphia, 1984, JB Lippincott.
5. McInnes J: *Clark's positioning in radiography,* ed 9, vol 1, Chicago, 1973, Mosby–Year Book.
6. Muller ME: *The hip.* In Evarts CM, editor: *Surgery of the musculoskeletal system,* vol 3, New York, 1983, Churchill Livingstone.

INDEX

5000591072